GENETIC
DISTANCE

GENETIC DISTANCE

Compiled by

James F. Crow
and
Carter Denniston

Genetics Laboratory
University of Wisconsin
Madison, Wisconsin

PLENUM PRESS · NEW YORK AND LONDON

Library of Congress Cataloging in Publication Data

Main entry under title:

Genetic distance.

"Papers presented at a workshop during the fourth International Congress of Human Genetics held in Paris, September,
1971."
Includes bibliographies and index.
1. Gene frequency—Congresses. 2. Human population genetics—Congresses. I. Crow, James F., ed. II. Denniston, Carter,
ed. III. International Congress of Human Genetics, 4th, Paris,
1971. [DNLM: 1. Genetics, Human—Congresses. 2. Genetics,
Population—Congresses. QH431 W923g 1971]
QH455.G46   573.2'1'3   74-23683

ISBN-13:978-1-4684-2141-5   e-ISBN-13: 978-1-4684-2139-2
DOI: 10.1007/978-1-4684-2139-2

Papers presented at a Workshop during the Fourth International
Congress of Human Genetics held in Paris, September, 1971

© 1974 Plenum Press, New York

softcover reprint of the hardcover 1st edition 1974

A Division of Plenum Publishing Corporation
227 West 17th Street, New York, N.Y. 10011

United Kingdom edition published by Plenum Press, London
A Division of Plenum Publishing Company, Ltd.
4a Lower John Street, London, W1R 3PD, England

PREFACE

Included in the program of The Fourth International Congress of Human Genetics, held in Paris on September 6-11, 1971, was a Workshop of Genetic Distance. This session, organized by Newton E. Morton, included several papers and a discussion under the general chairmanship of James F. Crow. Many of the participants and members of the audience asked at the time that the papers be printed so as to have a permanent record. It has not been practical to record the discussion, but all the papers originally presented are included in this volume.

The idea behind the Workshop was to take advantage of the large number of people who would be attending the Congress and bring together those who were interested in human population structure and measures of genetic distance.

The emphasis was on methodology; the number of methods almost equals the number of persons working in the field. The Workshop offered an opportunity to present and discuss the various procedures and review their accomplishments. The aim has been to have these papers either present the methods themselves, or give references as to where they can be found.

Some of the papers herein are exactly in the form originally presented at the Workshop, some are abbreviated versions, and others have been modified in the light of the discussions that took place. They have had a minimum of editorial treatment. They are reproduced here almost exactly as they were submitted by the authors, with only the minimum alterations required to fit the general format. We think this is preferable to editing the rather heterogeneous presentations into an artificial uniformity.

CONTENTS

INDICATORS OF GENETIC DISTANCE

I. Barrai

*Human Genetics Unit, World Health Organization
Geneva, Switzerland*

In recent years, considerable attention has been devoted to measuring the genetic distance between populations, and several indices of distance have been proposed and used.

Basically, one population is thought of as located at a point in a gene frequency space with dimensions depending on the number of loci and alleles under consideration, so that a Euclidean or an angular distance between any two populations in this space may be computed (WRIGHT 1968).

Among others, SANGHVI and STEINBERG and their co-workers have used variants of the Euclidean distance to represent genetic differences between populations (BALAKRISHNAN and SANGHVI 1968, STEINBERG et al. 1966). CAVALLI-SFORZA and his co-workers (1969) have preferred mainly the angular transformation, on the grounds that its sampling variance is independent of gene frequencies in a wide range from approximately 5% to 95%. The functional dependence of these indicators of genetic distance on geographic distance has not been investigated.

A functional relationship between genetic similarity and geographic distance has been postulated by MALECOT (1966) and applied by MORTON and his co-workers (YASUDA and MORTON 1966) to several bodies of data. The genetic similarity is expressed as a kinship coefficient, which measures the probability that two alleles drawn at random from two populations are identical by descent.

1

Since a relation between indicators of genetic distance and inbreeding indicators has begun to emerge—for example, CAVALLI-SFORZA has found a proportionality between the square root of the Wahlund coefficient of inbreeding and his measure of genetic distance—it seemed appropriate to study the variation of several indicators of genetic distance as a function of geographic distance, and compare them with the variation of the kinship coefficient. For simplicity, data which may approximate an unilocal two allele system were used.

LIVINGSTONE (1967) has published extensive data on β-thalassemia; the material used in this work is taken from his books and is represented by the frequency of osmotic fragility is 83 villages in Sardinia. The frequency of osmotic resistance was considered indicative of a heterozygous state for β-thalassemia, and a gene frequency for the thalassemia gene was calculated for each village. The linear distance between villages was then measured, and the values of the indices of genetic distance and kinship were then calculated for groups of villages at the same distance. The unit of geographical distance was five kilometers.

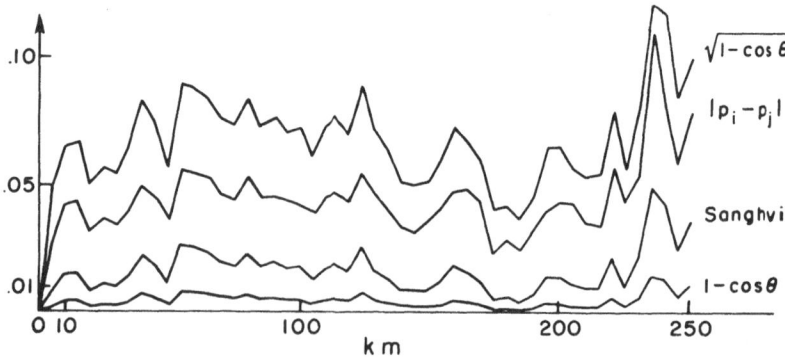

FIGURE 1. Variation of indices of genetic distance as a function of geographic distance. One locus, two alleles.

The results of the analysis are given in FIGURE 1.
Whatever the limitations inherent in the type of data used,
one may observe that all the indicators tested have the same
properties; in fact, they seem to differ only by a scale
factor.

The genetic distance measured by the indicators increases
with geographic distance; the trend is not so evident for
distances above one hundred kilometers, probably because
altitudinal variations between villages, clinal effects and
sample size interfere with the phenomenon.

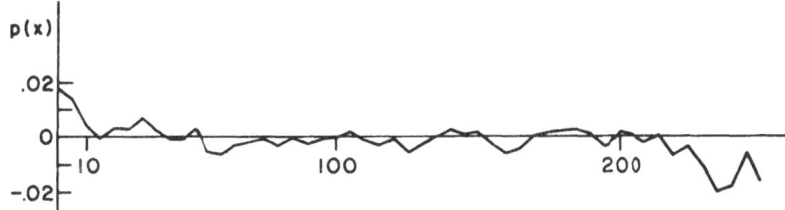

FIGURE 2.   Variation of the kinship coefficient ϕ_x with
geographic distance (kilometers) for β-thalassemia in 83
Sardinian villages.

The variation of the kinship coefficient is given in
FIGURE 2.   The variation in kinship is strikingly similar to
the variation in genetic distance, but it has an opposite
sense.   Clearly there is a simple relationship between indicators of genetic distance and kinship coefficient, so that
it might be desirable to express genetic distance as an explicit function of kinship.

SUMMARY

The variation of indicators of genetic distance and kinship as a function of geographic distance is investigated,
using data on the distribution of β-thalassemia in the island
of Sardinia.

The variation is practically the same for all indicators of genetic distance.

LITERATURE CITED

BALAKRISHNAN, V. and L. D. SANGHVI. 1968. Distance between populations on the basis of attribute data. *Biometrics* 24:859-865.
CAVALLI-SFORZA, L. L. 1969. Human Diversity. *Proc. XII Intern. Congr. Genetics* 3:405-416.
LIVINGSTONE, F. 1967. *Abnormal Hemoglobins in Human Populations*. Aldine, Chicago.
MALECOT, G. 1966. Identical loci and relationship. *Proc. Vth Berkeley Symp. Math. Statist. Probabil., Vol. 4*, pp. 317-332.
STEINBERG, A. G. et al. 1966. Genetic studies on an inbred human isolate.

MEASUREMENT OF DISTANCE AND PROPINQUITY IN ANTHROPOLOGICAL STUDIES

MORRIS GOODMAN and GABRIEL W. LASKER

Department of Anatomy, Wayne State University School of Medicine, Detroit, Michigan 48201

Various kinds of distance are significant in anthropological studies. We define *genetic distance* between two individuals (or between two populations) as the proportion of nonmatching nucleotide bases at homologous nucleotide sites between the genomes of two individuals (or of two populations). Since the matching nucleotide bases in these genomes are by and large the same by reason of descent from a common ancestor, genetic distance is also a measure of genetic or phylogenetic divergence. As yet there is no way to determine the nucleotide sequences of entire genomes, but there are data which can be used to deduce the nucleotide sequences of individual genes and to sample the proportion of nonmatching nucleotide sites (i.e. the genetic distance) between genomes.

Data for measuring genetic distance and hence for estimating genetic and phylogenetic divergence of genes, come from comparing the amino acid sequences of homologous polypeptide chains. Depending upon the proteins of polypeptide chains investigated, these sequences can help decipher genetic relationships among organisms at all taxonomic levels, from individual differences within populations to differences between the animal and plant kingdoms. The most common event

---

We acknowledge support by grants from the Systematic Biology and U. S. - Japan Cooperative Science Programs of the National Science Foundation and Grant HDO 4815 from the Public Health Service.

5

in the ongoing process of evolution, the point mutation, often
produces a difference in an amino acid residue in the sequences of proteins. The sequences are therefore an excellent
method for estimating the distance created by establishment
of point mutations in pedigrees and populations.

Other types of biological tests give results that can
also be used for distance measurements. The sequence homology between DNA from two sources (HOYER et al. 1964, MARTIN
and HOYER 1967, KOHNE 1970) can be determined by complemen-
tary base pairing. The correspondence of protein antigenic
sites in different organisms can be evaluated by immunodiffusion comparisons in modified Ouchterlony plates (GOODMAN
1963a, 1963b, 1967, 1968; GOODMAN and MOORE 1971). This
method works well in depicting genetic relatedness at the
intermediate (generic through subordinal) taxonomic levels.
Allelic frequency data, gathered by typing the polymorphic
forms of enzymes and other proteins, usually by electrophoretic techniques, can measure in a rough way the genetic distances among individuals or populations at the lower (infra-
generic) levels of species and within species. Typing blood
cell isoantigens and serum protein allotypes by immunological
procedures can permit the calculation of gene frequency differences in the same way.

CONSTRUCTION OF GENE AND ANIMAL PHYLOGENIES

FROM AMINO ACID SEQUENCE DATA

Amino acid sequence data permitting man to be compared
to other mammals are available for cytochrome C, alpha and
beta chains of hemoglobin, fibrinopeptides A and B, and carbonic anhydrase I. These yield information on differences in
about 550 codons in the corresponding gene loci, usable for
assessing the phylogenetic relationships of man. A phylogenetic tree is a tree-like diagram which depicts the phylogenetic relationships for a group of species, subpopulations,
or genes. The units whose phylogeny is being depicted (consisting of the original species, subpopulations, or genes for
which the necessary data are available and their reconstructed
most recent common ancestors) are called "Taxonomic Units".
For the construction of a gene phylogenetic tree, one considers
the amino acid sequences (or corresponding codon sequences) in
a set of polypeptide chains to be homologous if it can be in-
ferred that they descended from a common gene ancestor. One
makes this inference if each member of the set has a sequence

similar to other members of the set. For example, by broad
definition of genetic homology, all vertebrate myoglobin and
alpha and beta hemoglobin chains are homologs related by their
descent from a common gene ancestor which presumably existed
in the first vertebrates. However, by a more restricted
definition of genetic homology employed for constructing
animal phylogenetic trees, the alpha chains in mammalian
hemoglobins are a set of homologs; the beta chains are another
set.

Once it is decided which protein chains are homologous,
the amino acid positions in these chains are aligned so as
to maximize codon homologies throughout the set. Then minimum
mutation distances for every pairwise comparison of aligned
amino acid sequences can be calculated by the approach of
FITCH and MARGOLIASH (1967). This approach, based on the
genetic code, gives for each amino acid pair the minimum number of nucleotides that would need to be changed in order to
convert a codon for one amino acid into a codon for the other.
Since there are three nucleotide positions in each codon, up
to three nucleotide exchanges can be detected over each pair
of amino acids.

Using such minimum mutation distances among aligned
amino acid sequences, one can form a phylogenetic tree by a
calculating procedure based on the "divergence hypothesis",
that the more ancient is the common ancestor for a pair of
taxonomic units, the greater is the genetic distance between
that pair of taxonomic units. MOORE (1971) has shown that
the unweighted pair group method of SOKAL and MICHENER (1958)
is suitable, under this hypothesis, for constructing phylogenetic trees. Recent evidence (reviewed by KING and JUKES
1969) that there are many nucleotide positions in codon sequences at which selectively neutral mutations can accumulate,
suggests that, in their descent from a common ancestor, gene
lineages are especially likely to conform to the divergence
hypothesis. In other words, genes drift further and further
apart with the passage of time.

However, one might conjecture (GOODMAN 1961, 1962, 1965)
that more mutations were neutral to natural selection in the
primordial genes of ancestral organisms than in the descendant
genes of today's advanced organisms. Consider, for example,
earlier and later evolutionary stages in the descent of the
globin genes. While the original or prototype single-chained
globin probably had a heme-binding site and a tertiary struc-

ture similar to today's globins, it probably did not have the
array of functioning sites needed for subunit combination, for
binding diphosphoglycerate, for allosteric modulation of structure to promote the Bohr effect, or for combining with haptoglobin. Until the globin surface sites had acquired these
useful functions through evolution, many mutations affecting
them were presumably neutral to natural selection. But, after
acquiring functions, formerly neutral sites became fixed in
different lineages, since further mutations in such sites
would be detrimental and be selected against. From this, it
can be deduced that the primordial globin genes evolved at a
more rapid rate than the later globin genes of vertebrates.
To generalize, after higher levels of molecular organization
had evolved in living systems, increasing numbers and kinds
of functional restraints might well have decreased the number
of mutations accepted by natural selection, causing molecular
evolution at many gene loci to decelerate in higher organisms.

Thus, nonuniformity in evolutionary rates can be expected
between gene lineages. If these nonuniformities are sufficiently marked, the condition specified in MOORE's model for
the divergence hypothesis is not always exactly met by real
data. It has been observed that gene phylogenetic trees of
various cytochrome Cs, globin chains, and fibrinopeptides
calculated by the unweighted pair group method depict slightly
incorrect relationships for occasional branches, judged by
notions based on the fossil record. These trees can be altered
by trying alternative phylogenetic trees in a way which makes
efficient use of the mutation distance information to estimate
how the lineages descending from a common ancestor vary among
themselves with respect to rate of mutational change (FITCH
and MARGOLIASH 1967, BARNABAS et al. 1971, GOODMAN et al.
1971). From the original minimum mutation distance data, a
mutation length is calculated between each pair of adjacent
units. Then for each pair of units the mutation lengths are
summed through the shortest route of adjacent nodes connecting
the two units. Such reconstructed mutation distances are compared to the original distances based on the least number of
codon differences needed to account for the differences in
amino acid residues of homologous sites. The phylogenetic
tree with the least total deviation between reconstructed and
original mutation distances is considered the closest approximation to the correct phylogenetic tree. Experience so far
suggests that such trees resemble an animal phylogeny derived
from the fossil record.

Another approach to estimating the correct phylogenetic tree for a set of homologous polypeptide chains is to reconstruct the most plausible codon sequences of the past species as they were at the nodes of branching on a given tree in such a way that they give the smallest number of nucleotide substitutions over the entire tree. Once one has a method for reconstructing such parsimonious ancestral sequences, the next step is to find the most parsimonious tree, i.e. the particular branching arrangement which gives fewer nucleotide substitutions over the entire tree than any other topology would give (see FITCH 1971, also unpublished) and MOORE (elsewhere in this volume). Firstly, it has to be proven that the procedure chosen to construct from a set of known contemporary amino acid sequences and from a given estimated phylogenetic tree of these sequences gives the most parsimonious ancestral codon sequence, i.e. that no other ancestral sequence which could have been chosen gives fewer nucleotide changes. Secondly, it has to be shown that using the criterion of minimum nucleotide change over the entire tree provides a truer criterion reflecting biological reality than others which might be used to choose the "best" tree such as the unweighted pair group method.

Despite these theoretical restrictions on specific methods, it is fair to say that the construction of gene phylogenetic trees from amino acid sequence data by procedures of the type discussed above should contribute significantly to our knowledge of genetic evolution. One of the findings (BARNABAS et al. 1971) revealed by the phylogenetic tree of mammalian beta-like hemoglobin chains and the corresponding mutation distance matrix of these chains concerns the rates at which duplicated beta genes evolve compared to their parent genes. More mutational change is observed in the descent of the ceboid monkey delta globin gene line than in the descent of the ceboid beta line after these lines originated from their common gene ancestor (presumably in the early Anthropoidea); yet among the same ceboid monkeys, less divergence in delta genes than in beta genes occurred. Similar examples of a more rapid initial evolution of duplicated genes are provided by bovid beta (BARNABAS et al. 1971), and possibly by gamma hemoglobin chains (GOODMAN et al. 1971). These patterns of mutational distances suggest the following interpretation. After the beta gene duplications occurred, mutations accumulated freely at the duplicated loci until certain fortuitous mutations resulted in the emergence of new beta proteins with useful functions. Then natural selection not

only caused these particular advantageous mutant genes to
spread rapidly through the populations in which they occurred
but also drastically slowed their further evolution.

In attempting to represent animal phylogenies from the
gene phylogenetic trees, one notes that while two genes, each
in a different animal, can never have a common ancestor more
recent in time than the common animal ancestor of the two
animals, they can have a common gene ancestor more ancient
in time than the most recent common animal ancestor. Thus,
e.g., the topology of the mammalian beta globin gene tree
reveals that the separation between human delta chain and
gorilla, chimpanzee, or human beta chain is more ancient than
the separation between any two of these hominoid beta chains.
On the other hand, the separation in time between mouse beta
and human delta is no greater than between mouse beta and
human beta, since the primate beta duplication which produced
the ancestor of the human delta gene occurred after the animal
ancestors of mouse and man had separated from each other. For
an animal phylogenetic tree, the mutation distance between man
and gorilla would be determined solely by the human beta and
gorilla beta comparison, whereas the mutation distance between
man and mouse would best be the average from the comparisons of
mouse beta with both human beta and human delta.

The apparent ability of particular gene phylogenies, such
as the alpha globin one, to depict the relationships of animal
species has a marked grade or organismal aspect to it. The
evidence is clear that globin gene duplications are constantly
occurring. No doubt each genome contains a population of
nucleotide sequences descended from these duplicative events.
Yet natural selection apparently ensures a relative stability
of genetic regulatory mechanisms and structural gene expression in related lines of mammals. The genes which are active
in alpha globin chain synthesis in two animal species appear
in most cases as though they were direct descendants of the
same gene in the most recent ancestor of the two species.
Other sets of protein homologs, even the more evolutionarily
labile beta-like globin chains, also tend to show this relationship in which gene phylogenies coincide with animal
species phylogenies. The fact that a good degree of evolutionary stability exists with respect to those particular
structural loci which are ordinarily active in protein synthesis in related organisms makes it possible to use proteins
to construct phylogenetic trees of animals.

These animal trees have been constructed from the sequences of alpha and beta-like globins, fibrinopeptides, cytochrome C, and carbonic anhydrase I, and from combinations of these (GOODMAN et al. 1971, also unpublished data). The trees consistently demonstrate, in agreement with extensive immunodiffusion results (e.g., GOODMAN et al. 1970, GOODMAN and MOORE 1971) and also with DNA sequence homology data (HOYER et al. 1964, MARTIN and HOYER 1967, KOHNE 1970), an extremely close genetic relationship of the African apes to man. They also show a much higher degree of genetic correspondence between the two main branches of the Catarrhini, the cercopithecoids and hominoids, than between the bovine and caprine branches in the family Bovidae. The percent mutational divergence from combined sequence data between hominoids and cercopithecoids is less than half the divergence found between caprines and bovines. Yet, the paleontological evidence points to the caprine-bovine branching point being in the late Miocene and clearly no earlier than Miocene times, i.e., this branching occurred in the range of 15 to 25 million years ago. On the other hand, the cercopithecoid-hominoid split is placed by paleontologists back in the middle Eocene and not later than Oligocene times, i.e., from about 45 to 30 million years ago. Thus, for the particular amino acid sequences examined (which represent from 1000 to 1500 nucleotide positions or mutational sites), molecular evolution was much slower in the catarrhine primates than in the bovids. Furthermore, on using paleontologically estimated dating times for the nodes or branching points on the amino acid sequence phylogenetic trees, to calculate the rates of nucleotide change in the descending lineages, the results indicate that molecular evolution decelerated in the higher primates. Similar conclusions have been drawn with respect to DNA evolution (KOHNE 1970), and the possibility was emphasized that steadily increasing generation lengths may have been an important parameter (GOODMAN 1962, KOHNE 1970) in slowing molecular evolution in the descent of man during the Tertiary epoch.

Although such a phenomenon can be related to a decrease on a per year basis of the actual mutation rate on the assumption that the occurrence of fresh mutations depends on the DNA replication cycle, the role of natural selection should not be ignored. The development during the Tertiary epoch of such organs as the placenta and the cerebral neocortex in the eutherian mammals was probably accompanied by new biochemical adaptations and an overall increase in the level of molecular

organization within man's progenitors. The added functional
restraints brought about by such an increase in molecular
complexity could also increase the chances that any fresh
mutations would be detrimental to natural selection. An
immunological mechanism could further restrict the degree
of genetic variability within higher primate populations,
for the hemochorial placenta (with its intimate apposition
of fetal and maternal blood streams) and the long gestation
period increases the risk to the fetus from maternal immuni-
zation to fetal allotypes.

GENETIC PROPINQUITY AND MATING DISTANCE

WITHIN THE HUMAN SPECIES

In contrast to the measurements of distance used between
species, within the human species it is more customary to
measure similarity. Such measurements of similarity or propinquity are the reciprocal of distance. Genetic propinquity
may be defined as the degree of genetic similarity between
specific individuals or groups. Thus within a population it
would be measured by comparing genetic similarity between two
specified individuals with the mean similarity between random
individuals in the group. Measurement of propinquity in a
pedigree is called the coefficient of kinship.

Within a sexually reproducing species, the propinquity
between the two parents of individuals is of special genetic
interest. WRIGHT's (1922) coefficient of inbreeding, F,
measures the likelihood that two alleles of an individual are
identical by descent from a common ancestor. This is possible
only when the two parents are consanguineous and had the ancestor in common. Since the likelihood of a particular autosomal allele being transmitted is 1/2 at each generation,
$F = (1/2)^N$ where N is the number of steps back to the common
ancestor in both lines of descent. For the individual, the
value of F is the sum of the F's derived for each common ancestor. For the population, F is the mean of the F's for all
its individuals.

Since WRIGHT's F in human populations is calculated from
pedigrees, it usually spans only a few generations. The
greater the number of generations, the more likely are errors
of incorrect ascription of paternity. Furthermore, since one
cannot calculate inbreeding occurring in generations prior to
those included in the pedigree, only minimum estimates of the

coefficients of inbreeding can be derived from pedigrees.
One can, of course, assume constant or other rates of consanguineous unions for some span of generations for which
data are lacking and calculate corresponding values for inbreeding. Besides the possibility of errors in the assumed
inbreeding rates, which are likely to increase with the number
of generations, there are other sources of error. Thus, as
larger numbers of generations intervene, the effect of descent
from common ancestors is modified by the additional likelihood
of mutation and of differential selection in each generation.
These effects are proportional to the number of generations
in the maternal plus paternal lines of descent from common
ancestors. Even with the same estimated amount of inbreeding,
the larger the number of generations, the less is the likelihood of homozygosity by reason of the common descent.

For large spans of time, efforts to use historic records
of "invasions" and other population movements often prove to
be fruitless exercises in circular reasoning from the known
degree of biological propinquity of the subsequent populations
to the earlier ones. There are virtually no satisfactory quantitative data on the genetic significance of ancient migrations.
Measurements of genetic (or phenotypic) distance or propinquity
are the only ones available. They do not necessarily represent
the same thing as coefficients of kinship, however. One should
not be surprised by the poor fit of measures of genetic distance to those of common ancestry (kinship) based on linguistic
or cultural criteria (GILES et al. 1966, 1970, SALZANO 1968,
FITCH and NEEL 1969). Using genetic distance measurements as
a way of estimating degrees of common origin ignores adaptive
evolution and the consequent convergent and divergent processes
(LIVINGSTONE 1971). This difficulty can be avoided if the
measures of distance are not taken as an end in themselves but
are used to measure the evolutionary processes.

Another approach to the whole question of distance is to
study the geographic distance at which human beings mate and
the relation of this to inbreeding. If one asks informants,
"Where was your mother born?", "Where was your father born?",
and studies the distribution curves of measurements between
the two sites, it is seen that the curves are characteristic
of the socio-cultural status of the populations. These curves
are skewed and sometimes irregular because human populations
are not very homogeneously distributed. The curves are usually
represented by their medians or the square root of the mean
squared distances. Peasant populations have very short

breeding distances of this kind. The circle within which members of peasant communities characteristically marry is smaller in area than that of other kinds of people (LASKER unpublished data for Paracho and Mitla, Mexico, the Italian Alps, and for four places in Peru). If the measurement is in terms of the number of people within a circle with a radius of the median distance, the populations of hunters and gatherers are smaller than those of peasants, however. Thus, when they were discovered in 1818, the Arctic Eskimos of Thule, Greenland, ranged some distance up and down the coast but did not know that any other human beings existed; yet, they consisted of only 250-300 people by later censuses (MALAURIE et al. 1952).

There is, unfortunately for ease of calculation, a third dimension in human breeding distance: *social distance*. Perhaps it would be best to state this in the plural; there are higher order dimensions: social distances. Caste, class, and culture (above all, perhaps, religious affiliation) influence mate selection. The highest inbreeding coefficients for human populations occur on tiny islands far from other inhabited places--such as Tristan da Cunha (ROBERTS 1969), the Wellesley Islands (SIMMONS et al. 1962, 1964), Pitcairn (SHAPIRO 1929), and Saint-Barthelemy (BENOIST 1964)--and in religious isolates (subpopulations cut off from the large populations among whom they live by differences in religious practices) such as the Samaritans (BONNE 1963), the Habbanite Jews (BONNE et al. manuscript), Hutterites (MANGE 1964), Old Order Amish (CROSS and McKUSICK 1970), and German Baptist Brethern (GLASS et al. 1952). High mountain valleys are sometimes almost as endog-amous: Saas (HUSSELS 1969) and Canton Ticino (HULSE 1957) in Switzerland; Bellino, Italy (CHIARELLI and others unpublished); Paracho (LASKER 1954), Tlascala and San Pablo del Monte, Mexico (HALBERSTEIN and CRAWFORD 1971); and the New Guinea Highlands (GILES et al. 1966, 1970). Fishermen of San Jose, Peru (LASKER and KAPLAN 1964), Ramah Navaho herders (SPUHLER and KLUCKHOHN 1953) and farmers of Monsefu and Reque, Peru (LASKER and KAPLAN 1964), the Parma Valley in Italy (CAVALLI-SFORZA 1963), the Dinka (ROBERTS 1956) Coniagui and Bassari (LESTRANGE 1950, 1951), and Bedik (GOMILA 1971) of Africa provide some other instances of varying degrees of mating distances. YASUDA and MORTON (1967) have shown that, in some instances at least, mating distance is associated with inbreeding or the coeffi-cient of kinship.

Mating distances measured in kilometers have also been

compared with biological heterogeneity. The usual biological
scale is that of differences in gene frequencies for red cell
antigens (blood groups). Among the above examples, such
studies show local differentiation among Tristanites, two
groups of Wellesley Islanders, the people of St. Barthelemy,
Samaritans, Habbanites, Hutterites, German Baptist Brethern,
Tlascalans, several New Guinea populations and the villages
of the Parma Valley. These are what have been called "rip-
ples in the gene pool". The discontinuities may be small or
large but they appear as escarpments rather than gradual
clines on maps of gene frequency distributions.

     Even urban communities show some short breeding distances.
DUNN and DUNN (1957) found both endogamy and distinctive gene
frequencies in the Jewish quarter of Rome. The significance
of simple distance may be attenuated in the city, however,
because of social distances. Individuals seek as mates members of their social group rather than their own neighbors.
C. S. COON (1966) once asked how one can draw clines for skin
color in New York. The same problem would occur for any polymorphism. The bases for choice of mates in cities are hardly
at all geographic; they are largely in terms of ethnicity and
economic status.

     In such situations, very indirect methods may be helpful.
CROW and MANGE (1965) have suggested, and YASUDA and MORTON
(1967), MORTON and HUSSELS (1970), HUSSELS (1969) and SWEDLUNG
(1971) among others, have applied data on surnames in distance
studies. Isonymy, the likelihood of a surname to recur independently in two (affinal) lines in a pedigree, can be used to
calculate an index comparable to the inbreeding coefficient.
On the assumption of monophyletic names and their stability
through time, the recurrence of the same surname in affinal
relatives is a result of inbreeding. Isonymy occurs at about
the frequency one would expect if it were the result of random
mating between individuals in the community; that is, the sum
of products of the frequency of each surname in males by that
of the same name in females divided by the square of the number
of pairs. To the extent that the frequency of observed isonymy
is approximately that which would occur from random mating is
general (some unpublished data for Mexico are in agreement in
this respect with that published by LASKER 1969 for Peru),
lists of surnames can be used to measure the likelihood of
isonymy and can be related to measurements of genetic distance.

     In urban studies, data on surname frequencies and isonymy

offer an approach to breeding distance even though this is
not amenable to direct methods (LASKER 1970, T. REED personal
communication). At least the ethnic factor in social distance
may be partially controlled in this way.

Differences in the frequencies of surnames between males
and females are related to the matrimonial residency practices
(MORTON and HUSSELS 1970). For instance, under a system of
exogamous patrilocal marriage, the surnames of married males
in the community will be fewer and more frequent than those
of their wives. The frequency with which surnames are held
in common between communities can also be used as a measure
of recent common origins (JUBERG et al. in press, FRIEDL unpublished). Studies of surnames can thus measure the extent
of such modes of migration as well as estimate the extent of
inbreeding.

We now know of many human polymorphisms. Some of these
yield genetic distances of men on a worldwide basis; for instance, MOURANT and his colleagues (1954, 1958) have surveyed
the blood groups, LIVINGSTONE (1967) the hemoglobins, KIRK
(1968) haptoglobin and GIBLETT (1969) other serum proteins.
Similar worldwide surveys or breeding distances or isonymy
are not available. One could, however, extrapolate from
known breeding distances to distribution of distances characteristic of the whole human species. To do so one would
first need to define the types of people of the world in
socio-economic terms: Western industrial workers, Asian
peasants, Arctic hunters, etc. Sample studies of breeding
practices of each type can be weighted according to the number
of each such kind of individuals to produce a distribution
curve or array of curves which would characterize the species.
To the extent that the world is undergoing predictable socio-
economic changes, one could project future curves of mating
distances and develop models for the prediction of rates of
gene flow and reduction in the steepness of gene frequency
clines. It is circular reasoning to try to use genetic distances to reconstruct the influence of historical population
movements on human differences. Rather as ARMELAGOS and VAN
GERVEN (1971) have emphasized, research into the genetic
effects of social and cultural practices requires assessment
of genetic distances and independent evaluation of the demographic and other socio-cultural influences that may be
involved.

The increase in genetic distance varies in rate during

Primate phylogeny. Furthermore, recent common origins are not necessarily reflected in close similarity in gene frequencies between human populations. The study of the processes involved is therefore necessary to help explain genetic diversity.

We thank Dr. G. William Moore for criticizing the manuscript.

LITERATURE CITED

ARMELAGOS, G. J. and D. VAN GERVEN. 1971. Current direction in physical anthropology: comment. *Newsletter of Am. Anthrop. Assoc.* 12(2):8.

BARNABAS, J., M. GOODMAN and G. W. MOORE. 1971. Evolution of hemoglobin in Primates and other therian mammals. *Comp. Biochem. Physiol.* 39:455-482.

BENOIST, J. 1964. Saint-Barthelemy: physical anthropology of an isolate. *Am. J. Phys. Anthrop.* 22:473-487.

BONNE, B. 1963. The Samaritans: A demographic study. *Human Biol.* 35:61-89.

BONNE, B., S. ASHBEL, G. BERLIN and A. TEL. (Manuscript). The Habbanite isolate. II. History, demography and mating patterns.

CAVALLI-SFORZA, L. L. 1963. Genetic drift for blood groups. In *The Genetics of Migrant and Isolate Populations*, edited by E. Goldschmit, Williams and Wilkins, Baltimore.

COON, C. S. 1966. The taxonomy of human variation. *Ann. N. Y. Acad. Sci.* 134:516-523.

CROSS, H. E. and V. A. McKUSICK. 1970. Amish demography. *Social Biol.* 17:83-101.

CROW, J. F. and A. P. MANGE. 1965. Measurement of inbreeding from the frequency of marriages between persons of the same surname. *Eugen. Quart.* 12:199-203.

DUNN, S. P. and L. C. DUNN. 1957. The Jewish community of Rome. *Sci. Amer.* 196(3):118-128.

FITCH, W. M. 1971. Toward defining the course of evolution: Minimum change for a specific tree topology. *Systematic Zool.* 20:406-416.

FITCH, W. M. and E. MARGOLIASH. 1967. Construction of phyletic trees. *Science* 155:279-284.

FITCH, W. M. and J. V. NEEL. 1969. The phylogenetic relationships of some Indian tribes of Central and South America.

Am. J. Hum. Genet. 21:384-397.

GIBLETT, E. R. 1969. *Genetic Markers in Human Blood.*
Blackwell, Scientific Publications, Oxford.

GILES, E., R. J. WALSH and M. A. BRADLEY. 1966. Micro-
evolution in New Guinea: the role of genetic drift.
Ann. N. Y. Acad. Sci. 134:655-665.

GILES, E., S. WYBER and R. J. WALSH. 1970. Micro-evolution
in New Guinea: additional evidence for genetic drift.
Archaeol. and Phys. Anthrop. Oceania 5:60-72.

GLASS, B., M. S. SACHS, E. F. JOHN and C. HESS. 1952.
Genetic drift in a religious isolate: an analysis of
the causes of variation in blood group and other gene
frequencies in a small population. *Am. Nat.* 86:145-159.

GOMILA, J. 1971. *Les Bedik Senegal oriental: barrieres
culturelles et heterogeneite biologique.* Presses de
l'Universite de Montreal.

GOODMAN, M. 1961. The role of immunochemical differences
in the phyletic development of human behavior. *Hum.
Biol.* 33:131-162.

GOODMAN, M. 1962. Evolution of the immunologic species
specificity of human serum proteins. *Hum. Biol.* 34:
104-150.

GOODMAN, M. 1963a. Serological analysis of the systematics
of recent hominoids. *Hum. Biol.* 35:377-436.

GOODMAN, M. 1963b. Man's place in the phylogeny of the
primates as reflected in serum proteins. In *Classification and Human Evolution,* edited by S. L. Washburn,
Viking Fund Publications in Anthropology, Chicago.

GOODMAN, M. 1965. The specificity of proteins and the
process of primate evolution. In *XII Colloquium on
Protides of the Biological Fluids,* edited by H. Peeters,
Elsevier Publishing Co., Amsterdam.

GOODMAN, M. 1967. Deciphering primate phylogeny from macromolecular specificities. *Am. J. Phys. Anthrop.* 26(2):
255-275.

GOODMAN, M. 1968. Evolution of the catarrhine primates at
the macromolecular level. *Primates in Med.* 1:10

GOODMAN, M. and G. W. MOORE. 1971. Immunodiffusion systematics of the Primates. I. The Catarrhini. *Systematic
Zool.* 20(1):19-62.

GOODMAN, M., G. W. MOORE, W. FARRIS and E. POULIK. 1970. The
evidence from genetically informative macromolecules on
the phylogenetic relationships of the chimpanzees. In
The Chimpanzee, Vol. 2, edited by G. H. Bourne, Karger,
New York, pp. 318-360.

GOODMAN, M., J. BARNABAS, G. MATSUDA and G. W. MOORE. 1971.

Molecular evolution in the descent of man. *Nature* 233: 604-613.

HALBERSTEIN, R. A. and M. H. CRAWFORD. 1971. A demographic comparison of Mestizo and Indian populations of Tlascala, Mexico. (manuscript)

HOYER, B. H., B. J. McCARTHY and E. T. BOLTON. 1964. A molecular approach to the systematics of higher organisms. *Science* 144:959-967.

HULSE, F. S. 1957. Exogamie et heterosis. *Arch. Suisse d'Anthrop. Gen.* 22:103-125.

HUSSELS, I. 1969. Genetic structure of Saas, a Swiss isolate. *Hum. Biol.* 41:469-479.

JUBERG, R. C., W. J. SCHULL, H. GERSHOWITZ and L. M. DAVIS. 1971. Blood group gene frequencies in an Amish deme of northern Indiana: comparison with other Amish demes. *Hum. Biol.* (in press).

KING, J. L. and T. H. JUKES. 1969. Non-Darwinian evolution. *Science* 164:788-798.

KIRK, R. L. 1968. The haptoglobin groups in man. In *Monographs in Human Genetics,* edited by L. Beckman and M. Hauge, Karger, New York.

KOHNE, D. E. 1970. Evolution of higher organisms DNA. *Quart. Rev. Biophys.* 3:327-375.

LASKER, G. W. 1954. Human evolution in contemporary communities. *Southwestern J. Anthrop.* 10:353-365.

LASKER, G. W. and B. A. KAPLAN. 1964. The coefficient of breeding isolation: population size, migration rates, and the possibilities for random genetic drift in six human communities in Northern Peru. *Hum. Biol.* 36: 327-338.

LASKER, G. W. 1969. Isonymy (Recurrence of the same surnames in affinal relatives): A comparison of rates calculated from pedigrees, grave markers, and death and birth registers. *Hum. Biol.* 41:309-321.

LASKER, G. W. 1970. Physical Anthropology: The search for general processes and principles. *Am. Anthrop.* 72:1-8.

LESTRANGE, M. 1950. La population de la region de Youkounkoun en Guinee Francais. *Population* 5:643-668.

LESTRANGE, M. 1951. Pour une methode socio-demographique. *J. Soc. Africanistes* 21:97-109.

LIVINGSTONE, F. B. 1967. *Abnormal Hemoglobins in Human Populations.* Aldine, Chicago.

LIVINGSTONE, F. B. 1971. Gene frequency differences in human populations: Some problems of analysis and interpreation. In *Anthropological Genetics,* edited by M. H. Crawford, Univ. New Mexico Press (in press).

MacMAHON, B. and J. C. FOLUSIAK. 1958. Leukemia and ABO
    blood group. *Am. J. Hum. Genet.* 10:287-293.
MALAURIE, J., L. TABAH and J. SUTTER. 1952. L'isolat
    esquimaux de Thule (Groenland). *Population* 7:675-692.
MANGE, A. P. 1964. Growth and inbreeding of a human
    isolate. *Hum. Biol.* 36:104-133.
MARTIN, M. A. and B. H. HOYER. 1967. Adenine plus thymine
    and guanine plus cytosine enriched fractions of animal
    DNA's as indicators of polynucleotide homologies. *J.
    Molec. Biol.* 27:113-129.
MOORE, G. W. 1971. A mathematical model for the construction
    of cladograms. Ph.D. Thesis, North Carolina State Univ.
MOORE, G. W. A counterexample to FITCH's method for maximum
    parsimony trees. [This volume.]
MORTON, N. E. and I. HUSSELS. 1970. Demography of inbreeding
    in Switzerland. *Hum. Biol.* 42:65-78.
MOURANT, A. E. 1954. *The Distribution of the Human Blood
    Groups.* Blackwell, Scientific Publications, Oxford.
MOURANT, A. E., A. C. KOPEC and K. DOMANIEWSKA-SOBCZAK. 1958.
    The ABO Blood Groups. C. C. Thomas, Springfield, Ill.
ROBERTS, D. F. 1956. A demographic study of a Dinka village.
    Hum. Biol. 28:323-349.
ROBERTS, D. F. 1969. Consanguineous marriages and calcula-
    tion of the genetic load. *Ann. Hum. Genet.* 32:407-410.
SALZANO, F. M. 1968. Intra- and inter-tribal genetic vari-
    ability in South American Indians. *Am. J. Phys. Anthrop.*
    28:183-190.
SHAPIRO, H. L. 1929. *Descendants of the Mutineers of the
    Bounty.* Bishop Museum, Honolulu.
SIMMONS, R. T., J. J. GRAYDON and N. B. TINDALE. 1964.
    Further blood group genetical studies of Australian
    Aborigines of Bentinck, Mornington and Forsyth Islands
    and the mainland Gulf of Carpentaria, together with fre-
    quencies for natives of the Western Desert, Western
    Australia. *Oceania* 35:66-80.
SIMMONS, R. T., N. B. TINDALE and J. B. BIRDSELL. 1962. A
    blood group genetical survey in Australian Aborigines of
    Bentinck, Mornington and Forsyth Islands, Gulf of Car-
    pentaria. *Am. J. Phys. Anthrop.* 20:303-320.
SOKAL, R. R. and C. D. MICHENER. 1958. A statistical method
    for evaluating systematic relationships. *Kansas Univ.
    Sci. Bull.* 38:1049
SPUHLER, J. N. and C. KLUCKHOHN. 1953. Inbreeding coeffi-
    cient of the Ramah Navaho population. *Hum. Biol.* 25:
    295-317.
SWEDLUNG, A. C. 1971. The genetic structure of an historical

population: A study of marriage and fertility in Old Deerfield, Massachusetts. Research Reports Number 7, Dept. Anthropology, Univ. Mass., Amherst.

WRIGHT, S. 1922. Coefficients of inbreeding and relationship. *Am. Naturalist* 56:330–338.

YASUDA, N. and N. E. MORTON. 1967. Studies on human population structure. In *Proc. IIIrd Intern. Congr. Human Genet.*, edited by J. F. Crow and J. V. Neel, Johns Hopkins Press, Baltimore.

GENEALOGIES ET DISTANCE ENTRE POPULATIONS

Albert Jacquard

*Institut National D'Etudes Demographiques
Paris*

LE CONCEPT DE "DISTANCE"

Définition d'une Distance

Caractériser un objet c'est, le plus souvent, énoncer une série de mesures; ainsi, un individu peut être caractérisé par ses mesures anthropométriques, une population par les fréquences des gènes présents en un locus.

Cet ensemble de mesures peut être considéré comme un vecteur $M \equiv (x_1 \ldots x_n)$.

Comparer deux objets de même nature consiste alors à calculer les écarts entre leurs mesures, autrement dit à déterminer un vecteur égal à la différence:

$$\Delta \equiv M_1 - M_2 \equiv [(x_{11} - x_{22}) \ldots (x_{1n} - x_{2n})]$$

Mais lorsque les mesures sont nombreuses, en pratique, dès qu'elles sont au nombre de 4 ou 5, l'esprit a du mal à les saisir dans leur ensemble et à donner une réponse à la simple question fondamentale "l'objet 1 est-il plus 'proche' de l'objet 2 ou de l'objet 3?". Pour répondre l'on est tenté de rechercher un indice synthétique, qui caractérisera, en un seul nombre, la "distance" entre les objets.

NOTE: Some of the material in this article also appears in Dr. Jacquard's book, <u>The Genetic Structure of Populations</u>, Springer-Verlag, 1973.

Mais le mot "distance" est ambigü; bien plus, il est
traître, car il évoque un concept qui fait partie de notre
expérience concrète, quotidienne, la "distance géographique",
mesurée dans l'espace euclidien où nous nous mouvons. Depuis
notre jeune âge, nous savons, grâce à Pythagore, que la distance $d(1,2)$ de deux points 1 et 2 est donnée par:

$$[d(1,2)]^2 = (x_1-x_2)^2 + (y_1-y_2)^2 + (z_1-z_2)^2 \qquad (1)$$

où x_1, y_1, z_1 sont les coordonnées du point 1 dans un système
d'axes orthogonaux et normés; cette relation peut s'exprimer,
en considérant l'ensemble des trois coordonnées du point 1
comme formant un vecteur vertical C_1, par l'égalité

$$[d(1,2)]^2 = (C_1-C_2)'(C_1-C_2) \qquad (2)$$

où C' est le transposé du vecteur C.

On pourrait évidemment, par analogie, définir une distance entre deux objets 1 et 2 caractérisés par n mesures en
utilisant une formule telle que (1) où la somme serait étendue
à ces n mesures; on se placerait ainsi dans un "espace à n
dimensions". Mais il est évident qu'une telle démarche est
risquée; de quel droit assimilons-nous ces mesures à des
coordonnées dans un espace orthonormé alors que, par exemple,
- s'il s'agit de mesures anthropométriques, les diverses
mesures sont corrélées entre elles, la connaissance de l'une
constituant une information sur l'autre,
-s'il s'agit de fréquences géniques, celles-ci sont liées par
la relation évidente

$$p_1 + p_2 + \ldots + p_n = 1 ?$$

En fait, définir une distance revient à remplacer n
nombres par un seul nombre, donc à perdre de l'information,
et comporte une part d'arbitraire considérable. Parmi les
distances possibles la "bonne" distance correspond simplement
à l'intuition que nous avons au sujet des objets mesurés ou
à l'usage que nous voulons faire des concepts de "proximité"
et d'"éloignement".

Avant tout, il n'est sans doute pas inutile de rappeler
ce qu'est la définition d'une distance:

Soit un ensemble E; une distance définie sur E est une

application, définie sur E × E et à valeurs dans R_+ (c'est à dire associant à chaque couple (i,j) d'éléments de E un nombre réel positif d(i,j)), telle que

$d(i,j) > 0$ si $i \neq j$

$d(i,i) = 0$

$d(i,j) = d(j,i)$

$d(i,j) \leq d(i,k) + d(k,j)$.

La dernière de ces conditions correspond dans le plan à l'"inégalité du triangle"; un côté est plus petit que la somme des deux autres.

Naturellement face à un ensemble, il est possible de construire autant de distances que l'on désire, chacune ayant des propriétés plus ou moins adaptées au problème que l'on veut étudier ou correspondant plus ou moins bien à l'objectif de l'étude. Avant de présenter une utilisation du concept de distance dans un problème génétique: l'évaluation à partir des généalogies de la rapidité d'évolution du patrimoine biologique d'un groupe, nous rappellerons la définition de distances dont l'usage est largement répandu: le "D²" de MAHALANOBIS, l'"Arc" de CAVALLI-SFORZA et EDWARDS, le "X²" de BENZECRI; ce rappel a surtout pour but de souligner le caractère arbitraire de la définition d'une distance.

Le "D²" de Mahalanobis

Considérons des objets caractérisés par n mesures; à l'objet i correspond le vecteur $X_i = (x_{i1}...x_{in})$; ainsi un individu peut être caractérisé par un certain nombre de mesures anthropométriques. En général, ces mesures ne sont pas indépendantes, leur relations réciproques sont exprimées par la matrice des variances et covariances S définie par

$$S \equiv E[(X-\overline{X})(X-\overline{X})']$$

Ainsi la taille d'un individu et la longueur de son bras sont des mesures qui, sans être rigoureusement liées, sont en étroites corrélation: il est évident qu'en définissant une distance qui tiendrait compte indépendamment de l'écart entre les tailles et de l'écart entre les longueur de bras, on utilise en quelque sorte deux fois la même information.

D'autre part, une différence de 1cm sur la longueur d'un doigt représente de toute évidence un écart ayant plus de signification qu' une différence de 1cm sur la taille, étant donnée la plus grande variabilité de celle-ci.

Pour se ramener au cas habituel d'un espace où il soit naturel d'appliquer le théorème de Pythagore, c'est à dire où l'on puisse définir la distance entre deux points correspondants aux ensembles de mesures M_1 et M_2 par la relation (2) il est normal de chercher de nouvelles mesures $y_1...y_n$ qui soient

- fonction linéaires des mesures initiales $x_1...x_n$,
- indépendantes entre elles,
- et dont les écart-types constituent les unités.

Autrement dit, nous avons à déterminer une matrice A, telle que les mesures Y définies par $Y = AX$ aient pour matrice de variance-covariance, la matrice unité:

$$E[(Y-\overline{Y})(Y-\overline{Y})'] = I \tag{3}$$

On sait que si la matrice des variances-covariances de X est S, celle de $Y = AX$ est ASA'; la condition (3) s'écrit donc:

$$ASA' = I$$

soit, en multipliant cette expression à gauche par A^{-1} et à droite par $(A')^{-1}$:

$$S = A^{-1}A'^{-1} = (A'A)^{-1}$$

ou

$$A'A = S^{-1} \tag{4}$$

Etant donnée la façon dont nous les avons choisies, les nouvelles mesures Y définissent un espace dans lequel, par analogie avec l'espace géographique repéré par des axes orthonormés, il est naturel de calculer la "distance" entre deux points en ayant recours à la relation de Pythagore, c'est à dire en écrivant:

$$D^2 = (Y_1-Y_2)'(Y_1-Y_2)$$

$$= (X_1-X_2)'A'A(X_1-X_2)$$

soit d'après (4):

$$D^2 = (X_1-X_2)'S^{-1}(X_1-X_2) \tag{5}$$

relation qui définit la "distance de Mahalanobis".

On sait que cette distance, introduite ici par une voie purement intuitive, peut résulter, dans le cas de variables aléatoires ayant une distribution normale, de la recherche d'une fonction discriminante permettant de classer des objets en populations; mais dans la démarche décrite ici nous n'avons eu nul besoin de préciser cette condition.

Dans le cas où les variables x_i sont non corrélées, c'est à dire où la matrice S est une matrice diagonale

$$S = \begin{vmatrix} V_1 & & 0 \\ & V_i & \\ 0 & & V_n \end{vmatrix}$$

on a évidemment

$$S^{-1} = \begin{vmatrix} 1/V_1 & & 0 \\ & 1/V_i & \\ 0 & & 1/V_n \end{vmatrix}$$

et la distance de MAHALANOBIS se ramène à

$$D^2 = \sum_i \frac{(x_{1i}-x_{2i})^2}{V_i} \tag{6}$$

Dans ce cas particulier, mais dans ce cas seulement, la distance D^2 est équivalente à celles proposées par PEARSON en 1921 (coefficient of racial likeness) ou par PENROSE en 1954 (C_H^2), distances utilisées très fréquemment, en raison de la facilité des calculs qu'elles nécessitent, mais abusivement du fait de l'irréalisme de la condition de non-corrélation.

Les "Arc" et "Chord" de CAVALLI-SFORZA et EDWARDS

Considérons des populations caractérisées par les proportions de n caractères mutuellement exclusifs manifestés
par les individus qui les composent; ces populations sont
des objets à chacun desquels correspond un vecteur

$$P_i = (p_{i_1} \cdots p_{in})$$

avec évidemment

$$\forall i \; \sum_k p_{ik} = 1 \tag{7}$$

Les p_{ik} peuvent être, par exemple, les proportions d'
individus ayant tel phénotype ou telle taille, ou les
fréquences des divers allèles $a_1 \ldots a_n$ présents en un certain
locus.

Les vecteurs P_i correspondent, dans un espace à n
dimensions, à des points se déplaçant sur la portion de plan
définie par

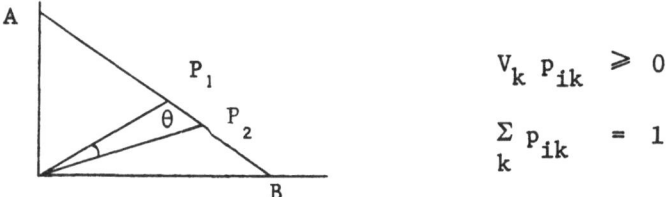

$$\forall_k \; p_{ik} \geqslant 0$$

$$\sum_k p_{ik} = 1$$

dans le cas où n = 2, il s'agit d'un segment de droite AB
situé dans le premier quadrant.

On peut songer à mesurer l'écart entre deux vecteurs
P_1 et P_2 par l'angle θ qu'ils forment, angle défini classi-
quement par la relation:

$$\cos \theta = \frac{\sum_i p_{1i} p_{2i}}{\left(\sum_i p_{1i}^2 \; \sum_i p_{2i}^2 \right)^{1/2}}$$

mais une telle mesure a l'inconvénient évident d'avoir une
sensibilité qui varie selon que les points P_1 et P_2 sont plus
ou moins proches d'une des extrémités de segment AB: un même
écart entre P_1 et P_2 sur la droite AB correspond à un angle
θ d'autant plus petit que P_1 et P_2 sont proches de A ou de B.

Pour éviter cet inconvénient, on peut effectuer un
changement de variable qui remplace les fréquences p_{ik} par
leurs racines carrés:

$$\pi_{ik} = \sqrt{p_{ik}}$$

la relation (7) devient (9)

$$\forall i \quad : \quad \sum_{k} \pi_{ik}^2 = 1$$

les vecteurs de coordonnées π_{ik} correspondent alors à des
points se déplaçant dans un espace à n dimensions, sur la
portion de l'hypersphère de rayon 1 située dans la zône où
toutes les coordonnées sont positives; dans le cas où n =
2, il s'agit de la portion AB du cercle de rayon 1 située
dans le premier quadrant.

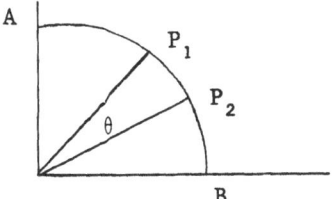

Si l'on mesure l'écart entre deux vecteurs par leur angle,
l'inconvénient d'une sensibilité variable est éliminé. Cet
angle est encore donné par une relation telle que (8) qui
devient, compte tenu de (9),

$$\cos \theta = \sum_{i} \pi_{1i}\pi_{2i} = \sum_{i} \sqrt{p_{1i}p_{2i}}$$

L'angle θ peut évidemment varier de 0 à $\pi/2$; CAVALLI-
SFORZA et EDWARDS ont préféré manipuler un paramètre variant
de 0 à 1, ils ont donc adopté comme distance

$$\text{Arc } (1,2) = \frac{2}{\pi} \text{ arc cos } \sum_i \sqrt{P_{1i}P_{2i}} \qquad (10)$$

(ce qui revient à exprimer θ en centaines de grades)

En vue de faciliter les problèmes d'estimation ces auteurs ont enfin souvent substitué à cette mesure, la longueur de la corde sous-tendant l'arc P_1P_2: on obtient facilement:

$$P_1P_2 = \sqrt{\sin^2 \theta + (1 - \cos \theta)^2} = \sqrt{2(1 - \cos \theta)}$$

Pour obtenir un paranètre variant dans des limites convenables ils ont à nouveau multiplié par $2/\pi$ et finalement défini la distance:

$$\text{Chord } (1,2) = \frac{2\sqrt{2}}{\pi} \sqrt{1 - \sum_i \sqrt{P_{1i}P_{2i}}} \qquad (11)$$

Il faut toutefois remarquer, à la suite de KIDD et COLL, que le coefficient $2/\pi$ est cette fois mal choisi puisque l'intervalle de variation de Chord est $(0, (2\sqrt{2})/\pi = 0,9003)$.

Généralisation: Considérons maintenant des populations caractérisées par les proportions de m séries de caractères mutuellement exclusifs (par exemple les fréquences alléliques constatées en divers locus).

En admettant que ces m séries sont indépendantes, on peut définir une distance globale dans l'espace des m mesures obtenues pour les différentes séries en appliquant simplement le théorème de Pythagore. CAVALLI-SFORZA et EDWARDS ont ainsi proposé de calculer la distance G_{12} définie par

$$[G_{(1,2)}]^2 = \sum_j [\text{Chord}_j (1,2)]^2$$

où la sommation est faite sur les m séries de proportions.

Le X^2 de BENZECRI

Considérons à nouveau des populations caractérisées par les proportions P_{ij} d'individus présentant le caractère j dans la population i et par leurs effectifs n_i; les caractères j sont mutuellement exclusifs, ce sont par exemple, les diverses

classes entre lesquelles on a réparti un caractère métrique,
ou les divers allèles présents en un locus.

Pour définir une "distance" nous partons de deux observations, qui correspondent à l'intuition que nous avons de la
proximité ou de l'éloignement des populations

1 - un écart entre les fréquences d'un même caractère dans
deux populations $P_{1j} - P_{2j}$ doit "peser" d'autant plus dans
le distance entre 1 et 2 que le caractère est plus rare dans
l'ensemble des populations, c'est à dire que la fréquence
moyenne: $P_{.j} = \Sigma_i n_i P_{ij} / \Sigma_i n_i$ est plus petite.

2 - si deux caractères j et k ont pour toutes les populations
des fréquences proportionnelles, c'est à dire si

$$Vi \; \frac{P_{ij}}{P_{ik}} = constante \; ,$$

on doit pouvoir remplacer ces deux caractères j et k par un seul
caractère l tel que:

$$P_{il} = P_{ij} + P_{ik}$$

Cette dernière condition correspond au fait que dans ce
cas, l'information fournie par le caractère k est toute entière
contenue dans celle fournie par le caractère j; il doit donc
être possible de les regrouper sans modifier les distances
entre populations.

On peut constater facilement que la distance euclidienne
classique définie par:

$$d^2(1,2) = \sum_j (P_{1j} - P_{2j})^2$$

ne satisfait pas cette condition, par contre une "distance de
X^2 définie par

$$X^2(1,2) = \sum_j \frac{(P_{1j} - P_{2j})^2}{P_{.j}} \tag{12}$$

la satisfait[1] et présente en outre l'avantage de pondérer
les écarts dans le sens de l'observation 1.

   Remarques. (a) Il faut bien noter que le vocable "distance du X^2" n'est utilisé ici qu'en raison de l'analogie
entre la relation (12) et la formule classique de définition
de la variable X^2; le paramètre X^2 n'est évidemment pas une
"variable X^2" puisque nous n'avons pas présenté les données
P_{ij} comme des variables aléatoires dotées d'une loi. (b)
Cette distance X^2 sert de base à la méthode d'"analyse des
correspondances" élaborée par J. P. BENZECRI, mais notre pro-
pos est seulement ici de l'utiliser pour caractériser des
distances entre populations. (c) Pour vérifier qu'il s'agit
bien d'une "distance", il suffit de remarquer que le changement de variable

$$Q_{ij} = \frac{P_{ij}}{\sqrt{P_{.j}}}$$

entraîne

$$X^2_{(1,2)} = \sum_j (Q_{1j} - Q_{2j})^2$$

X n'est donc autre que la distance euclidienne classique dans
l'espace de cette nouvelle variable Q. (d) SANGHVI (1953) a
proposé une mesure très voisine définie par:

---

[1] Si $P_{ij} = aP_{ik}$, $P_{.j} = aP_{.k}$, et $P_{il} = P_{ij} + P_{ik} = (1+a)P_{ik}$

d'où $\dfrac{(P_{1j} - P_{2j})^2}{P_{.j}} \dfrac{(P_{1k} - P_{2k})^2}{P_{.k}} = \dfrac{(P_{1k} - P_{2k})^2}{P_{.k}}(1+a)$

$$= \frac{[P_{1k}(1+a) - P_{2k}(1+a)]^2}{P_{.k}(1+a)}$$

$$= \frac{(P_{11} - P_{21})^2}{P_{.1}}$$

$$G^2 = \sum_j \frac{(r_{1j} - r_{2j})^2}{(r_{1j} + r_{2j})}$$

ce qui revient à utiliser une distance du X^2 basée non sur la moyenne des fréquences dans l'ensemble des populations, mais sur le double de la moyenne calculée dans le sous-ensemble des deux populations comparées. (e) Lorsque les populations sont caracterisées par plusieurs séries indépendantes de caractères mutuellement exclusifs, on peut, comme pour les mesures "chord", définir une distance globale par

$$X^2 = \sum_k X_k^2 \quad ,$$

où la sommation est étendue à l'ensemble des séries.

Exemple

Imaginons que 4 populations d'effectifs égaux soient caractérisées par les fréquences de 4 allèles présents en un certain locus; pour fixer les idées admettons que ces fréquences sont les suivantes:

Allèle Population	a_1	a_2	a_3	a_4
1	0	0	80	20
2	0	30	20	50
3	40	30	0	30
4	20	30	50	0
Moyenne	15	22,5	37,5	25

L'examen de ce tableau ne permet guère de se faire une opinion claire sur les proximités deux à deux de ces populations, sinon peut-être le fait que la population 1, qui ne possède que deux allèles, diffère plus sensiblement des autres.

a) On peut appliquer à ce tableau la méthode de D^2 de

MAHALANOBIS; il suffit de considérer que les fréquences moyennes des divers allèles constituent des "mesures" caractérisant les populations. Naturellement en raison de la relation

$$\sum_j P_{ij} = 1 \quad ,$$

il suffit de connaître 3 fréquences pour connaître la quatrième; celle-ci ne représente donc pas réellement une "information".

Si nous nous bornons aux 3 premiers allèles, la matrice des variances et covariances des fréquences est

$$S = 10^{-4} \begin{vmatrix} 275 & 112,5 & -312,5 \\ & 167,5 & -317,5 \\ & & 9,20 \end{vmatrix}$$

d'où

$$S^{-1} = \begin{vmatrix} 59,354 & -4,768 & 18,515 \\ & 173,011 & 58,088 \\ & & 37,206 \end{vmatrix}$$

et

$$D^2_{(1,2)} = (0 \quad -30 \quad 60) S^{-1} \begin{matrix} 0 \\ -30 \\ 60 \end{matrix} = 8,0533$$

On obtient ainsi

$$D(1,2) = 2,84$$
$$D(1,3) = 2,83$$
$$D(1,4) = 2,84$$
$$D(2,3) = 2,83$$
$$D(2,4) = 2,82$$
$$D(3,4) = 2,82$$

Toutes les populations sont donc pratiquement équidistantes.

b) La méthode de CAVALLI-SFORZA et EDWARDS donne

$$\cos \theta(1,2) = \sqrt{0,16} + \sqrt{0,10} = 0,7162$$

d'où

$\theta(1,2) = 0,492$	$\theta(2,3) = 0,517$
$\theta(1,3) = 0,842$	$\theta(2,4) = 0,577$
$\theta(1,4) = 0,564$	$\theta(3,4) = 0,604$

c) Le calcul de la distance X définie par la relation (12) aboutit à:

$X(1,2) = 13,1$	$X(2,3) = 11,6$
$X(1,3) = 17,9$	$X(2,4) = 12,3$
$X(1,4) = 10,3$	$X(3,4) = 11,4$

On voit que les résultats obtenus par ces diverses méthodes ne sont pas superposables, puisque l'ordre des distances n'est pas le même. Si l'on prend pour unité la distance entre les populations 1 et 2 qui est la plus petite
pour la mesure θ, la matrice des distances s'écrit:

	1	2	3		1	2	3
2	1				1		
pour θ: 3	1,71	1,05		pour X:	1,37	0,89	
4	1,15	1,17	1,23		0,80	0,95	0,87

Les populations 1 et 2, qui sont les plus proches selon
θ, sont, au contraire, relativement éloignées selon X puisque
seule la distance (1,3) est supérieure.

Cet exemple met bien en évidence la caractère arbitraire
d'une mesure de distance: le point essentiel est donc le
choix d'une distance adaptée à la question étudiée.

MESURE DE l'EVOLUTION A PARTIR DES GENEALOGIES

Probabilité d'origine des Gènes

Le plus souvent les évaluations de distances ont pour

objet de comparer des populations contemporaines; les données
de base sont des observations anthrométriques ou hémotypol-
ogiques; l'objectif est d'estimer la ressemblance ou la dis-
semblance des divers groupes et, éventuellement, de tracer un
arbre phylogénétique fournissant une explication satisfaisante
des écarts constatés.

Nous cherchons au contraire, dans ce qui suit, à comparer une même population avec elle-même au cours du temps; les
données sont les généalogies recueillies sur un nombre de générations aussi grand que possible; l'objectif est d'évaluer la
transformation du patrimoine génétique du groupe au cours des
générations.

Lorsque l'on dispose de généalogies, il est classique de
calculer le "coefficient moyen de consanguinité" défini comme
"la probabilité pour que les deux gènes d'un individu pris au
hasard soient identiques, c'est à dire soient la réplique d'un
même gène ancêtre."

Mais ce seul chiffre, malgré l'intérêt évident de sa signification biologique, en ce qui concerne notamment l'appauv-
rissement du patrimoine génétique, est un résumé bien insuf-
fisant des informations très riches contenues dans les généalogies. Celles-ci, en fournissant pour chaque individu la
liste de ses ancêtres , indiquent les chemins qu'ont pu par-
courir les gènes dont il est doté.

Pour chaque locus, chaque génôme comporte deux gènes qui
proviennent d'un ou de deux ancêtres parmi les 2^n (au plus)
qui constituent l'ascendance à la génération n. Il est évidemment impossible de préciser quels sont les ancêtres qui
ont effectivement fourni ces gènes; on peut seulement affecter
à chacun d'eux une probabilité d'être la source d'un de ces
deux gènes; comme dans la plupart des problèmes de génétique,
un recours au raisonnement probabiliste s'impose.

De façon précise, nous définissons comme "ancêtres in-
itiaux" ou "fondateurs" d'une population, les individus dont
nous ne connaissons ni le père ni la mère. Ces fondateurs
peuvent être classés en "ancêtres présents dans le groupe à
telle époque", "immigrants entrés dans le groupe à telle
époque", "immigrants provenant de telle origine", etc., de
façon à regrouper les résultats obtenus.

Lorsqu'un seul des parents est connu, nous convenons

d'attribuer une désignation arbitraire au parent inconnu, qui
est alors considéré comme l'un des "fondateurs".

Pour chaque individu i appartenant, ou ayant appartenu,
à la population, il est aisé de calculer, à partir des généalogies, la probabilité P_{ij} pour qu'un de ses gènes provienne du fondateur j. Ce calcul long et fastidieux peut-être
effectué rapidement par un calculateur électronique.

En regroupant l'ensemble des individus qui constituent
un sous-groupe G (par exemple, une génération) on obtient
l'ensemble O_G des probabilités d'origine des gènes constituant le patrimoine de ce sous-groupe. Cet ensemble O_G est la
traduction la plus fidèle de la signification biologique des
généalogies.

Exemple. Ce travail a été réalisé pour la tribu des
indiens Jicaques du Honduras créée il y a un siècle par 7
fondateurs et pour laquelle l'ensemble des généalogies ont
pu être reconstituées. On a trouvé, pour les 5 générations qui
se sont succédé, les probabilités d'origine ci-après:

Généra-tion	Effec-tif	Fondateurs							Immigrants		
		Leon	Fran-cisco	Cacia-na	Juan	Poli-naria	Pedro	Petro-na	Total	In-diens	Metis
1	7	143	143	143	143	143	143	143	1000	–	–
2	34	88	74	74	191	176	199	199	1000	–	–
3	176	66	78	78	167	151	208	208	957	43	–
4	247	54	68	68	162	146	195	195	888	81	31
5	101	24	31	31	132	126	129	129	602	186	212
Moyenne pondérée		55	66	66	160	146	187	187	867	82	51

On voit combien l'interprétation d'un tel tableau est
aisée. Deux faits apparaissent avec une particulière netteté:

-- la modification rapide des parts des divers fondateurs.
-- l'importance des gènes introduits par les immigrants.

Ce dernier point ne peut être révélé que par la voie
suivie ici; au contraire les statistiques classiques d'immigration, basées sur les nombres d'individus entrés dans la
tribu, peuvent faire croire que ce courant a été extrèmement
faible puisqu'il atteint à peine 4% de l'effectif total de

chaque génération. La raison de cet écart important est la
fertilité élevée des couples comportant un immigrant, qui a
accru considérablement leur part dans le patrimoine biologique transmis aux nouvelles générations.

Distance Entre Générations

Rapidité de l'évolution. Si dans deux générations suc-
cessives les probabilités d'origine des gènes sont différentes,
le patrimoine génétique de la population s'est déformé; les
gènes transmis par tel ancêtre fondateur ont pris une place
plus importante au détriment des gènes provenant de tel autre.
Ainsi dans le cas des Jicaques, les gènes de Leon qui repré-
sentaient 143% du patrimoine global de la génération 1, celle de la fondation du groupe, n'en représentent plus que 88%
dans la génération 2; simultanément la part des gènes de Juan
passe de 143% à 191%. Ces écarts résultent évidemment de la
dispersion des fécondités des couples et de la dispersion des
mortalités infantiles des diverses fratries.

Pour caractériser la transformation ainsi intervenue entre 2 générations, il est utile de définir une distance entre
les vecteurs "probabilités d'origine". Nous pouvons alors remarquer que, si les deux fondateurs formant un couple procréateur n'ont pas eu d'enfants autre que ceux de ce couple, les
probabilités d'origine les concernant sont définitivement
égales. Tel est le cas par exemple, chez les Jicaques, de
Francisco et Caciana d'une part, Pedro et Petrona d'autre
part. Il est clair que le tableau des données doit, compte-
tenu de cette remarque, pouvoir être simplifié en remplaçant
l'ensemble des 2 individus par le couple qu'ils forment; la
distance que nous avons à définir devrait ne pas être modifiée
par un tel regroupement.

Cette remarque nous incite à utiliser une distance telle
que le "X^2" qui n'est pas affecté par cette opération. Nous
adoptons donc pour mesurer l'écart entre les patrimoines géné-
tiques de deux générations g et g' paramètre $X(g,g')$ défini
par

$$\left[X_{(g,g')}\right]^2 = \sum_i \frac{(P_{ig} - P_{ig'})^2}{P_i} \tag{13}$$

où p_{ig} est la probabilité pour qu'un gène pris au hasard chez un individu de la génération g provienne du fondateur i, et p_i la moyenne de ces probabilités pour l'ensemble des générations (pondérée naturellement par leurs effectifs).

Dans le cas des Jicaques, on obtient:

$$X(1,2) = 15,6 \quad X(2,3) = 6,3 \quad X(3,4) = 6,7 \quad X(4,5) = 29,7 \; .$$

L'évolution, d'abord très rapide en raison de l'extrême faiblesse de l'effectif du groupe, s'est ensuite ralentie pendant deux générations avant de s'accélérer sous l'effet de l'invasion du patrimoine biologique du groupe par des gènes immigrés. (Insistons à nouveau sur le fait qu'il ne s'agit nullement d'une invasion du groupe par des individus immigrés, mais d'une diffusion plus large des gènes de ces immigrés favorisée par leur plus grande fécondité.)

CONCLUSION

Pour l'ethnologue, l'anthropologue, le démographe, une population est un ensemble d'individus, se renouvellant de génération en génération. Pour le généticien, une population est avant tout un ensemble de gènes se perpétuant identiques à eux-mêmes, malgré la diversité des hommes qui en sont porteurs; au-delà de l'apparence provisoire des êtres, il étudie la réalité biologique profonde du groupe: son patrimoine génétique.

La déformation progressive de ce patrimoine sous l'effet des actions sélectives du milieu, du comportement matrimonial et du comportement procréateur des individus, ou simplement sous l'effet du hasard peut être mesurée lorsque l'on connait l'ensemble des généalogies, autrement dit lorsque l'on possède pour tous les individus vivants ou morts, jusqu'à une certaine génération considérée comme "fondatrice", les triplets d'information: {identité de l'individu - identité de son père - identité de sa mère}.

La mesure de cette déformation nécessite la définition, obligatoirement arbitraire, d'une "distance"; il semble que, pour ce problème, une distance basée sur une métrique du X^2 soit particulièrement bien adaptée.

BIBLIOGRAPHIE

BALAKRISHNAN V. SANGHRI, L. D. 1968. Distance between populations on the basis of attribute data. *Biometrics* 24:859-865.
BENZECRI, J. P. Analyse des Correspondances. *I.S.U.P.*, Paris.
CAVALLI-SFORZA, L. L. et A. W. F. EDWARDS. 1967. Phylogenetic Analysis. Models and Estimation Procedures. *Am. J. Hum. Genet.* 19:233-257.
CHAPMAN, A. M. et A. M. JACQUARD. 1971. Un isolat d'Amérique Centrale, les Jicaques du Honduras. *Génétique et Population, INED, PUF*, Paris.
DEFRISE-GUSSENHOVER, E. 1967. Generalized Distance in Genetic Studies. *Acta Genetica* 17:275-288.
DUCIMETIERE, P. 1970. Les méthodes de la classification numérique. *Revue de Statistique Appliquée* 18-4 25.
KIDD, K. K. et L. A. L. SGARAMELLA-ZONTA. 1971 Phylogenetic Analysis Concepts and Methods. *Am. J. Hum. Genet.* 23: 235-252.
STEINBERG, G. A., H. K. BLEIBTREU, J. W. KURZYNSKI, A. O. MARTIN et E. M. KURCINSKI. 1966. In *Proc. Third. Int. Congress Hum. Genetics*, Chicago.

DISTANCE MEASURES FOR PHYLOGENETIC TREES

A. W. F. Edwards

Department of Medicine, University of Cambridge

REPRESENTATION OF DATA

In the treatment of statistical data it is important to distinguish between methods of *representation* and methods of *analysis*. Histograms and scatter diagrams, for example, provide means of representing data and are a useful preliminary to analysis; the use of logarithmic graph paper or of one of the many probability papers is similarly beneficial. It is not to be supposed that the mere plotting of points on gaussian probability paper constitutes an analysis, or that such a plot is only valid if the points are in fact normally distributed, for the very departure from normality may provide the stimulus for subsequent analysis.

Distance measures which have been proposed for use with phylogenetic trees have sometimes been criticized as a method of analysis. They were, however, never intended as a method of *analysis*, but only as a method of *representation* prior to analysis by the technique for estimating phylogenetic trees (e.g. those of CAVALLI-SFORZA and EDWARDS 1967, EDWARDS 1970). To criticize the transformation which leads to the distance measure described below for not being dependent on the observed correlations in gene frequency between populations is like criticizing a demographer for using logarithmic graph paper to study population growth, on the grounds that no actual population grows exponentially.

41

A DISTANCE MEASURE

Let p_i and p'_i be the gene frequencies of the ith allele at a k-allelic locus in each of two populations. Then EDWARDS (1971) has proposed the measure of genetic distance

$$\frac{4\sqrt{2}}{\pi}\sqrt{\frac{1 - \Sigma\sqrt{(p_i p'_i)}}{[1 + \Sigma\sqrt{(p_i/k)}][1 + \Sigma\sqrt{(p'_i/k)}]}}$$

gene substitutions, the sums being over i = 1, 2 ... k. Populations thus represented will lie in a Euclidean space of (k - 1) dimensions, and hence information from independent loci may be combined using Pythagoras' theorem.

The development of the above formula has been described recently elsewhere. EDWARDS (1972) has given a general account of the background to phylogenetic analysis, and EDWARDS and CAVALLI-SFORZA (1972) have considered, at greater length, the meaning of "distance" in a stochastic context. EDWARDS (1971) gives the full mathematical derivation of the above distance formula.

GRAPH PAPER

Populations characterized by gene frequencies at a tri-allelic locus may be graphed in two dimensions, and graph paper may thus be constructed which incorporates the desired transformation. Examples are given in EDWARDS (1971) and EDWARDS and CAVALLI-SFORZA (1972). It is of some interest that EDWARDS (1971) records finding some similar graph paper, apparently produced in R. A. FISHER's department about twenty years ago.

LITERATURE CITED

CAVALLI-SFORZA, L. L. and A. W. F. EDWARDS. 1967. Phylogenetic analysis; models and estimation procedures. *Evolution* 21:550-570; *Am. J. Hum. Genet.* 19:233-257.

EDWARDS, A. W. F. 1970. Estimation of the branch points of a branching diffusion process. *J. Roy. Stat. Soc. B.* 32:155-174.

EDWARDS, A. W. F. 1971. Distances between populations on

the basis of gene frequencies. *Biometrics* 27:873-881.
EDWARDS, A. W. F. 1972. Mathematical approaches to the
    study of human evolution. In *Mathematics in the
    Archaeological and Historical Sciences*, edited by
    D. G. KENDALL, R. HODSON and P. TAUTU, Edinburgh Uni-
    versity Press.
EDWARDS, A. W. F. and L. L. CAVALLI-SFORZA. 1972. Affin-
    ity as revealed by differences in gene frequencies.
    In *The Assessment of Population Affinities in Man*,
    edited by J. WEINER, Oxford: Clarendon Press.

THE ANALYSIS OF GENETIC VARIATION USING MIGRATION MATRICES

Walter Bodmer and L. L. Cavalli-Sforza

Genetics Laboratory, Department of Biochemistry, University of Oxford, Great Britain and Genetics Department, Stanford University Medical School, Stanford, California 94305

One of the main aims of the population geneticist is to try to account for observed variations in gene and genotype frequencies over both time and space. Most populations are distributed irregularly in any given geographic area. Population sizes are often small enough so that, when variation over a relatively small geographic area is considered, simple deterministic models to account for the observed genetic variation are unsatisfactory because they ignore fluctuations due to random genetic drift. Though population sizes may be small, it is, nevertheless, rare for any given population to be sufficiently isolated from all others so that migration can be neglected. Even quite low levels of migration between relatively isolated populations may have very significant effects in counteracting divergence between them due to random fluctuations. Models to account for genetic variation observed in restricted geographic areas must, therefore, take into account population subdivisions of the area being studied and rates of migration between these subdivisions.

Many models have been suggested for dealing with this problem. As is so often the case, only the simplest models are mathematically reasonably tractable but their application

The research reported in this paper was supported in part by grants from the National Science Foundation (GB29094), the National Institutes of Health (GM10452-09) and the United States Atomic Energy Commission (AT(04-3)-326 PA#33).

to the analysis of observations is very limited because of
their simplicity. Models directed at answering the question
of the relative importance of random genetic drift, mutation,
selection and migration in the determination of observed
genetic variation must include applicable representations of
observed migration patterns.

   Migration models generally fall into two main categories.
The first considers populations distributed discretely into
small groups, such as villages, towns or tribes, which may
for convenience be called colonies. The pattern of migration
between these colonies may then be defined. The simplest and
first example of such a model is SEWALL WRIGHT's (1931)
"Island Model". This refers to a single finite population
which has a constant rate of immigration from an infinitely
large outer population. The second category of models considers that the population is distributed continuously in
space and that migration is defined by a distribution which
gives the probability that an individual will move a given
distance from his place of birth before giving rise to offspring. Such models have been analyzed extensively by MALECOT
(1950) and by WRIGHT (1943) who has called this approach the
study of "isolation by distance".

   The island model has been extended to an infinite population, distributed in colonies of finite and equal size, which
exchange individuals with their immediate neighboring colonies
at a given rate. This model has been considered by MALECOT
(1950), and by KIMURA and WEISS (1964) who called it "the
steppingstone model". Major drawbacks of these models are
that they generally treat only the equilibrium situation, and
that they depend on the assumption that migration is isotropic;
namely, that the rate of migration from a colony to its neighbors is independent of the position of that colony in the
population. Such an assumption is clearly incompatible with
most observed migration patterns, which may be quite irregular.

   Rates of migration in human populations can be estimated
with reasonable precision, especially when the populations are
subdivided into discrete well-defined colonies. We have suggested (BODMER and CAVALLI-SFORZA 1968) a method of analysis
which tries to make the best possible use of observed data on
migration among a group of colonies. This model has been
called a "migration matrix model", since the pattern of migration between the colonies can be defined in the form of a
matrix. Our main aim here is to review this model and its

applications.

It has been reemphasized by MORTON and co-workers that
a closely analogous approach was developed by MALECOT in a
paper which appeared in 1950 in the *Annales Mathematiques de
la Faculte des Sciences de Lyon*. This paper which fore-
shadowed many of the results later obtained by KIMURA and
WEISS (1964) and BODMER and CAVALLI-SFORZA (1968) is unfortunately not readily accessible and appears to have been
largely overlooked until quite recently. Migration matrices
have also been used in a few other genetic situations (see
ROBERTS and HIORNS 1962 and HIORNS et al. 1969). An approach
similar to that we shall discuss was published independently
by C. A. B. SMITH (1969). Recently, a series of papers has
also been published by MARUYAMA and MARUYAMA and KIMURA following essentially the same approach that we outlined in 1968
(see KIMURA and OHTA 1971).

MIGRATION MATRICES

Given that a population is clearly subdivided into a
number of discrete colonies, a migration matrix in its simplest form is a matrix whose elements are the numbers of
children born in colony i (rows) of parents who are born in
colony j (columns). In some cases where migration varies
with respect to sex, separate matrices can be constructed
for fathers and mothers, but in practice one can usually work
with the sum of these two matrices. The migration matrix
may, of course, change from one generation to the next.
Provided the matrix for each generation is known, the model
which we have analyzed can take this into account. It is,
of course, rare in human populations that migration matrices
for more than two successive generations are available.
Clearly, in many parts of the world, migration patterns have
been changing rapidly as a result of changes in communication
and means of transport, and this must limit the applicability
of any approach to studying patterns of genetic variation in
such situations. In some cases where written records give
migration information for past generations, it is possible
to check whether patterns of migration have been changing and
to what extent they have changed.

There is also another check on the consistency of a
given migration matrix with the observed population sizes of
the various colonies. Thus, if a migration matrix has re-

mained constant over a number of generations, it can be used
to predict the relative population sizes of the various colonies involved. The prediction depends upon the fact that
the forward migration matrix (in which the elements of the
observed matrix are normalized so that the sums of columns
are equal to one and so that the matrix represents the probability that individuals born in colony j go to colony i)
can be used to predict the expected change in colony sizes
from one generation to the next. Thus, if

$$\mathbf{n}_0 = (n_1, n_2, \ldots n_k)$$

is the (arbitrary) vector of population sizes at time t =
0, the expected composition of the population in the next
generation is given by

$$\mathbf{n}_1 = \mathbf{n}_0 \mathbf{M}_F \qquad (1)$$

where $\mathbf{M}_F$ is the forward migration matrix. After t generations
the expected population size will therefore be given by

$$\mathbf{n}_t = \mathbf{n}_0 \mathbf{M}_F^t \qquad (2)$$

on the assumption that the migration matrix has remained constant during this time. After a sufficiently large interval
of time, t, the vector $\mathbf{n}_t$ will converge to an equilibrium
value that can be predicted from the convergence of powers
of the forward migration matrix, and is independent of the
initial vector $\mathbf{n}_0$.

Three examples using these approaches to test the stability of migration patterns, give results as follows:

1. A migration matrix for a series of villages in the
upper Parma Valley has been obtained from data averaged over
the last three hundred years, a time when little change in
the patterns of migration has taken place. The expected composition of the population given by powering the forward
migration matrix is in good agreement with the observed relative sizes of the various villages (CAVALLI-SFORZA and ZEI
unpublished observations).

2. MALCOLM and others have obtained the migration matrix
for a series of clans of a tribe called the Bundis in New

Guinea. Their data refer to a large section of the tribe,
which was converted to Catholicism some 50 years ago. In
this case, clans rather than villages are taken as the population subunits for the construction of the migration matrix,
as these seem to be the more stable population groupings.
The villages which now exist have largely been created under
the influence of the Australian authorities in order to sim-
plify the administration of the tribes. The clan structure,
however, remained largely untouched by this geographic re-
distribution. With respect to this data, as in the previous
case, the relative clan sizes are predicted very well from
the powers of the migration matrix (TABLE I). This is remark-

TABLE I

NUMBER OF INDIVIDUALS IN BUNDI CLANS, OBSERVED AND EXPECTED

ON THE BASIS OF DEMOGRAPHIC EQUILIBRIUM COMPUTED FROM INTERNAL

MIGRATION MATRICES (FROM MALCOLM et al. 1971)

| | Number of | Individuals |
Clan	Observed	Expected
Aranam	43	42.5
Biyom	152	94.5
Bundi	228	124.8
Doakai	168	177.5
Emegari	297	378.4
Gegeru	857	772.6
Guyebi	290	235.9
Inau	91	160.2
Karisogo	548	892.0
Konarigim	48	51.9
Koroma	149	157.4
Mendi	740	613.6
Nombri	503	383.3
Tigina	93	79.5
Yandakari	594	645.2

able in view of the small population sizes, and hence the
relatively low precision of the migration matrix. MALCOLM
et al. (1971) have used a Monte Carlo approach to see to what
extent the differences between the observed relative sizes
and those expected based on the migration matrix could be due

to errors in the determination of the migration matrix due to
small population size. Their conclusions are that the differences are well within sampling error (see TABLE I).

3. The third example of the application of migration
matrices is to the Pygmies of the Central African Republic.
In this case, groups of villages rather than single villages
were considered as the population units. Pygmies live in
small camps so that it seemed reasonable to combine several
camps into a single unit. In this case, the comparison between observed relative population sizes and those expected
from the migration matrix was poor. This may be because it
is known that the Pygmies are receded into the forest as the
forest is being further exploited and destroyed. The migration matrix results suggest that some areas may soon be de-
populated of Pygmies unless present trends in migration change
(CAVALLI-SFORZA et al., unpublished).

PREDICTION OF GENETIC VARIATION USING MIGRATION MATRICES

The model proposed by BODMER and CAVALLI-SFORZA (1968)
uses migration matrices to generate a matrix of the variances
and covariances of gene frequencies for all the colonies that
are being studied. This model uses the backward migration matrix in which the elements of rows (rather than the columns)
are normalized so that their sum is 1. The terms of the backward matrix give the probabilities M_{ij} that a child born in
the ith colony comes from parents born in the ith colony.
The model assumes that two alleles, A and a, are segregating
at a single locus in each colony and that time is discrete,
being measured in generations. Within each colony, mating
takes place at random. It is further assumed that in each
generation a proportion α_i of the individuals in the ith colony
come from an external population with a constant A gene frequency of x_i. The α_i and x_i can be taken to represent the
total effect of all stabilizing factors, such as migration
from the outside, mutation and linearized effects of selection.
It can be shown that the expected gene frequencies in generation n, $p_i^{(n)}$ are given in terms of the frequencies in the
previous generation by the following equation:

$$p_i^{(n)} = \sum_{j=1}^{k} (1 - \alpha_i) M_{ij} p_j^{(n-1)} + \alpha_i x_i \qquad (3)$$

where k is the total number of colonies. When the values of x_i are unknown (as is usually the case), they are often taken to be a constant. It can be shown that this does not have much effect on the gene frequency variances and covariances.

Random sampling variation from generation to generation, namely, random genetic drift, is introduced by assuming that the actual gene frequency in the ith colony in the nth generation is the result of a binomial sample of size $2N_i$ (the number of genes in the ith colony), with expected gene frequency $p_i^{(n)}$ as given by (3). The aim is then to predict the variances and covariances of the gene frequencies in the colonies at any given time n. The algebra involved is greatly simplified by introducing the angular transformation of gene frequencies. This has the well-known advantage of making the variance of gene frequencies, which is a binomial variance, independent of the value of the gene frequency itself. This is an approximation which is only valid provided the gene frequencies are not too near zero or 1. In practice, as suggested by FISHER, who first proposed the angular transformation as a practical measure, simulation experiments have shown that the approximation matches the theoretical results reasonably well, at least in the range of gene frequencies between .05 and .95 (See BODMER and CAVALLI-SFORZA 1968.) Based on the assumption of the validity of the angualr transformation, it can be shown that the variances and covariances of the angular values $\theta_i^{(n)}$ of the gene frequencies in the nth generation are given approximately by the following equations:

$$V(\theta_i^{(n)}) = \frac{1}{8} \left[\frac{1}{N_i} + \sum_{j=1}^{n-1} \frac{1}{N_j} \sum_{r=1}^{n-1} (m_{ij}^{(r)})^2 \right] \qquad (4)$$

$$\mathrm{Cov}(\theta_i^{(n)}, \theta_j^{(n)}) = \frac{1}{8} \sum_{\ell=1}^{k} \frac{1}{N_\ell} \sum_{r=1}^{n-1} (m_{i\ell}^{(r)} m_{j\ell}^{(r)}) \qquad (5)$$

Variances of angular values can be transformed approximately into Wahlund variances $[\theta^2/\bar{p}(1 - \bar{p})]$ by multiplication by the factor 4.

Here N_i is the population size of the ith colony and $m_{ij}^{(r)}$ is the ijth term of the rth power of the modified migration matrix whose terms are given by

$$(1 - \alpha_i)M_{ij}$$

The variances and covariances given by (4) and (5) can be
calculated numerically given the values of N_i, α_i, and the
migration matrix, M_{ij}. In a few cases, it has been possible
to obtain simple analytical results for simplified migration
matrices, such as those which describe migration between adjacent colonies arranged in a circular pattern. These analytical results have been shown to correspond (with a small
approximation) to the results obtained by KIMURA and WEISS
(1964) for their linear stepping-stone model when the number
of colonies tends to infinity.

The variances and covariances given by (4) and (5) correspond to what would be expected from repeated realizations of
the whole process of the model as defined above, namely, by
binomial sampling imposed on (3). In practice, any set of
observations on gene frequencies corresponds to only a single
observation in time, so that only the variance in gene frequencies between the colonies at this point in time can be
used to match theory with observation. It is possible to obtain expressions for this expected variance in the gene frequencies between the various colonies in terms of the results
given by (4) and (5). This is the quantity which must be used
for comparison of the expected results of the theory with observations.

In any infinite population, in the absence of stabilizing
forces such as mutation or selection, the ultimate fate of any
allele is either fixation or extinction. It can be shown,
however, that provided at least one or more of the colonies
is subject to a linear stabilizing force, as represented by
the parameters α_i in our model, fixation or extinction for the
population as a whole are avoided. This parameter α_i is, in
fact, critical to the comparison of the model with observations. Given that it incorporates at least the effects of
migration from colonies outside those being directly considered, the question can reasonably be asked whether the observed variations match those expected on the basis of the
model. In this case, it can presumably be assumed that differential selection of one sort or another is not required to
explain a given observed set of variations in gene frequencies.

Differences in the values of the α's for different colonies can, of course, be made to incorporate the effects of differential selection or migration from the outside for the various colonies.

In calculating the observed variation in gene frequencies between a given set of colonies, it is very important that the sampling variance of the gene frequency estimates by eliminated from the observed variance of the gene frequencies. This may be a difficult problem, because gene frequency estimates are often made from populations in which individuals are interrelated in complicated ways (see ROBERTSON 1951, CAVALLI-SFORZA and BODMER 1971, MATESSI and JAYAKAR, unpublished observations). The use of covariances of the gene frequencies between the colonies, in principle, could remove this problem. However, when covariances between all pairs of colonies are considered, it is necessary to average these in some way and this introduces assumptions of isotropy with respect to migration. In addition, to obtain such average covariances, data from each colony are used a number of times and this duplication of information casts some doubt on the validity of the application of standard tests of significance to comparisons of the covariances.

COMPARISON OF OBSERVATION WITH THEORY

A number of comparisons have now been made of observations on gene frequency variation among a given group of colonies and expectations based on the migration matrix model. The observations are usually based on estimates of gene frequencies for a variety of blood groups and other polymorphisms. The expectations are calculated from a knowledge of the population sizes suitably corrected to give "effective population sizes" (see CAVALLI-SFORZA and BODMER 1971) and the migration patterns defined by a migration matrix, together with the all important alpha values for migration from the outside, as already discussed. The development of the migration matrix approach was stimulated by the analysis of data from the upper Parma Valley for which, as already mentioned, extensive migration data could be collected. Unfortunately, however, the available demographic records have not so far given rise to a satisfactory estimate of the alpha values. Preliminary calculations using the migration matrix model and given in TABLE II have been based on α values which may be in error. Another problem in the data from the Parma Valley has been connected with the

TABLE II

OBSERVED AND EXPECTED VARIATIONS IN GENE FREQUENCY

Population	Observed variance	Variance based on computer simulation	Equilibrium variance based on migration matrices
Parma Valley (Italy)	$.036^{(1)}$	$.0109^{(2)}$	$.0116^{(2)}$
Guatemalan Indians	$.0154\pm.0016^{(3)}$	---	$.021^{(3)}$
Bundi of New Guinea	$.008^{(4)}$	---	$.002^{(4)}$
Pygmies of the Central African Republic	$.0103-.0239^{(5)}$	---	$.005^{(5)}$
Makiritare Indians	$.0588\pm.0211^{(6)}$	---	$.0265\pm.0100^{(6)}$

All variances are standardized to correspond to Wahlund gene
frequency variances ($f = \sigma^2_p/pq$) and are averages for a variety of blood groups and other polymorphisms.

References: (1) CAVALLI-SFORZA et al. 1964. This value is
                   too high mostly because of bias upwards of
                   the method for estimation. Improved values
                   are being obtained.
             (2) CAVALLI-SFORZA and ZEI 1967, CAVALLI-SFORZA
                   et al. 1964.
             (3) CANN et al. (in press) The above data are
                   more complete, and figures slightly differ-
                   ent from those used by CAVALLI-SFORZA and
                   BODMER 1971.
             (4) MALCOLM et al. 1971. Observed variance not
                   significantly different from zero.
             (5) CAVALLI-SFORZA (in press). Range of esti-
                   mates refers to different estimation meth-
                   ods used.
             (6) NEEL and WARD 1970. Computation by
                   D. Wagener (unpublished).

statistical difficulties involved in the calculations of gene
frequency variances already mentioned. Preliminary results
indicate that the observed variance given in Table II was
computed by a method which can give rise to an upward bias
of as much as a factor of 2. In view of these problems, it
is perhaps not surprising that the estimate of the observed
variance of gene frequencies is higher, by a factor of three,
than that predicted by the migration matrix approach (see
Table II, first line). The migration matrix results could,
however, be compared with results obtained from a relatively
complete simulation of the population, as described by
CAVALLI-SFORZA and ZEI (1967), following an approach similar
to that also used by MACCLUER (1967). The artificial population simulated on the computer used the same migration matrix
as was used in the calculation of the variance based on the
migration matrix model and the results obtained are quite comparable (see Table II, line one). It is interesting to note
that the computer simulation of the population takes into account statistical variations in the rate of migration between
colonies. This factor is not taken into account by the migration matrix model nor, so far as we are aware, by any of the
other models which have been proposed for the analysis of gene
frequency variation. The agreement between the results from
the computer simulation and the migration matrix approach for
the upper Parma Valley population suggests that stochastic variation in migration rates is not an important source of variation in gene frequencies between a group of populations. Some
approaches to taking account of variation in migration rates
have recently been suggested by CANNINGS (unpublished).

Other comparisons of observations with the migration
matrix approach have been made for the Bundi tribes in New
Guinea (MALCOLM et al. 1971), for the Guatemalan Indians
around Lake Atitlan (CANN, unpublished), for the Pygmies of
the Central African Republic (CAVALLI-SFORZA, et al. 1969),
and for the Makiritare Indians (WARD and NEEL 1970).

Deviations between observed and expected variances
should be viewed in the light of difficulties connected with
the estimation of variance of gene frequencies. When examined with a variety of methods as e.g. for the Pygmy data,
observed variance changes by more than a factor of 2. The
standard errors of observed variances, estimated for instance
on the basis of the variation over 13 different loci for the
Makiritare Indians, are large and give an idea of the expec-

tedly low precision of variance estimates. Other sources of
error are inherent in the sampling error of the frequencies
of migrants in the migration matrices themselves. The standard error of the expected variance for the Makiritare Indians is obtained from the variation between $V(\Theta)$ values from
four migration matrices given by WARD and NEEL (1970). In
view of the statistical difficulties and high sampling errors,
the observed and expected values should be considered in substantial agreement. The collection of much more data in analogous situations should help in reaching more satisfactory
conclusions than are possible today.

These results suggest that when migration patterns and
population sizes of selected present day populations are taken
into account adequately, and when a study is limited to a fairly well defined and restricted geographical area, most, if not
all, of the observed variation in gene frequencies can be accounted for without allowing for differential or stabilizing
natural selection. This does not, of course, exclude the possibility that there is differential (disruptive) or stabilizing selection (heterosis), which is not sufficiently large in
magnitude to be detected. In addition, it must be emphasized
that all these studies have been restricted to relatively homogeneous areas from an ecological point of view. It is, of
course, less likely that differential or stabilizing selection
with respect to such populations will be found than for studies
made with a more dispersed set of populations. Thus, for example, studies of variation in polymorphic gene grequencies
between major racial groups do suggest the existence of selective effects (see CAVALLI-SFORZA 1966, CAVALLI-SFORZA 1971,
LEWONTIN and KRAKAUER, 1973).

An important feature of the migration matrix model is
that it does not assume that populations are in equilibrium
with respect to gene frequency variation. Thus, in principle, it allows the possibility of estimating the time that
may be taken to reach an equilibrium in the gene frequency
variances from a given hypothetical starting point. This
time will be a function of the parameters of the migration
matrix and of the α values, as well as, of the population
sizes. For example, in the case of the Guatemalan Indians,
the time needed to reach equilibrium is comparatively large
because of the very low rates of migration from one village
to another. This should lead to an observed variation in
gene frequencies which is smaller than that expected at equi-

librium from the migration matrix approach. On the other hand,
in the Parma Valley, the time needed to reach equilibrium is
expected to be of the order of 10 - 20 generations because
of a relatively high rate of migration between the villages
of the Valley. This time appears to be sufficient, based on
the demographic data that we have on migration patterns, for
one to expect that gene frequency variances should have been
at their equilibrium values.

APPLICATION TO SOME HYPOTHETICAL MIGRATION PATTERNS

     Some insight into the effects of variation in the para-
meters of the model and, for example, on problems such as the
effect of dimensionality on the variation in gene frequencies,
can be obtained by studying the consequences of the migration
matrix model with simple hypothetical migration patterns. As
already mentioned, in some cases, such as migration between
neighboring colonies arranged on a circle, complete analytical
solutions for the variances and covariances can be obtained.
These results can be compared with higher dimensional migration patterns, such as migration among colonies arranged on
a torus or at the vertices of a regular icosahedron. In all
cases we have found that there is very little effect of the
number of dimensions, either on the rate of approach to equilibrium or on the equilibrium variance of the gene frequencies.
This is in contrast to a much greater effect of dimensionality on gene frequency variances expected from the continuous
model. This difference may have something to do with the differences in the definition of dimensionality in discrete and
continuous models. In going from one to two dimensions in a
continuous model, the number of directions in which there is
opportunity for migration is increased infinitely, while for
discrete models the number of opportunities changes by no more
than a factor of 2 for each dimension.

     Other problems investigated previously (see BODMER and
CAVALLI-SFORZA 1968) included studies on the variation of
covariances and correlations with distance during the approach
to equilibrium. The theory developed by MALECOT (1950) and
by KIMURA and WEISS (1964) predicted that, at equilibrium,
gene frequency covariances and correlations should vary
exponentially with distance. The migration matrix model can
be used to establish how long it takes to approach the

exponential relation between gene frequency correlations
and distance. With migration between colonies arranged in
a 6 x 6 lattice, such an exponential relationship may in
fact never be valid. It is, in practice, unlikely that observed data could easily resolve deviations of gene frequency
covariances and correlations from the expected exponential
relationships. Departures from such a simple exponential
relationship may also be caused by nonhomogeneous migration
from the outside, namely, by differences in the alpha values
between the various colonies.

                              DISCUSSION

     IMAIZUMI and others (1970) favor the use of kinship co-
efficients as defined by MALECOT (1950), rather than gene
frequency variances as we have used them. These two sets of
quantities are, of course, closely related although they are
not identical. All the analytical approaches proposed so far,
seem to involve some element of approximation which is at
least comparable to that implied by our use of the angular
transformation. It should, however, be emphasized that estimates of kinship based, for example, on pedigrees (especially
if these refer to only a few generations) may give values which
are too far removed from the requirements of the theory for
them to be applicable.

     It is clear that the migration matrix approach itself is
still only an approximation to reality, though we do suggest
that it may be a better approximation than that provided by
some of the other methods that have, so far, been used to explain gene frequency variation. A major requirement for the
application of the migration matrix method is an estimate of
the migration matrix itself. A further limitation is that
the size of the migration matrix which can be handled by
available computers is, so far at least, not more than 40 or
50. It is, however, always possible, and perhaps even advis-
able from a biological point of view, to subdivide matrices
and analyze subregions separately. It is also possible to
combine rows and columns of the matrix so as to obtain a
matrix of lower rank. Comparisons between these various
analyses can be very useful and instructive. Difficulties
may, of course, also be encountered with highly mobile populations in which it is difficult or even impossible to define
population groups or areas. This difficulty has been emphasized
by WARD and NEEL (1970) for the Makiritare, where new groups

often seem to be formed by fission or fusion of preexisting groups. However, the results we have presented here would suggest that even in these cases it might still be worth trying to compare the consequences of the migration matrix approach with the observations.

SUMMARY

A brief outline of the migration matrix approach to the study of the variation in gene frequency between a defined set of populations has been given. Some examples of the application of this approach to comparison with observations on gene frequency variance have been discussed. It appears that migration matrices make it possible to take into account, in a more realistic way, observed migration patterns between populations. (Details of the analytical results discussed in this paper will be found in BODMER and CAVALLI-SFORZA 1968). The agreement between observed and expected gene frequency variances indicates that random genetic drift is probably the major cause of variation in gene frequencies among groups of villages or population units which are located in relatively restricted geographical areas, namely, to what might generally be called microgeographic differentiation. Further accumulation of data along the lines suggested here will help in clarifying the picture that emerges from the initial application of the method.

LITERATURE CITED

BODMER, W. and L. L. CAVALLI-SFORZA. 1968. A migration matrix model for the study of random genetic drift. *Genetics* 59:565-592.

CAVALLI-SFORZA, L. L. 1972. Pygmies, an example of hunters-gatherers, and genetic consequences for man of domestication of plants and animals. *IV Int. Congr. Human Genetics, Paris, Proceedings, 1971*. In press.

CAVALLI-SFORZA, L. L. 1966. Population structure and human evolution. *Proc. Roy. Soc. B.* 164:362-379.

CAVALLI-SFORZA, L. L., I. BARRAI and A. W. F. EDWARDS. 1964. Analysis of Human Evolution under random genetic drift. *Cold Spring Harbor Symposia on Quantitative Biology* 24:9-20.

CAVALLI-SFORZA, L. L. and W. BODMER. 1971. *The Genetics of Human Populations*, W. H. Freeman, San Francisco.

CAVALLI-SFORZA, L. L. and G. ZEI. 1967. Experiments with
    an artificial population. *Proc. Third Int. Congr.
    Hum. Genet.* The Johns Hopkins Press, Baltimore,
    pp. 473-478.
CAVALLI-SFORZA, L. L., L. A. ZONTA, F. NUZZO, L. BERNINI,
    W. W. W. DEJONG, P. MEERA KHAN, A. K. RAY, L. N. WENT,
    M. SINISCALCO, L. E. NIJENHUIS, E. VANLOGHEM and G.
    MODIANO. 1969. Studies on African Pygmies. I. A
    pilot investigation of Babinga Pygmies in the Central
    African Republic (with an analysis of Genetic distances).
    Amer. J. Hum. Genet. 21:252-274.
HIORNS, R. W., G. A. HARRISON, A. J. BOYCE and C. F.
    KUCHEMANN. 1969. A mathematical analysis of the ef-
    fects of movement on the relatedness between popula-
    tions. *Ann. Hum. Genet.* 32:237-250.
IMAIZUMI, Y., N. E. MORTON and D. E. HARRIS. 1970. Isola-
    tion by distance in artificial populations. *Genetics*
    66:569-582.
KIMURA, M. and T. OHTA. 1971. Protein polymorphism as a
    phase of molecular evolution. *Nature* 229:467-489.
KIMURA, M. and G. H. WEISS. 1964. The stepping stone model
    of population structure and the decrease of genetic cor-
    relation with distance. *Genetics* 49:561-576.
LEWONTIN, R. C. and J. KRAKAUER. 1973. Distribution of gene
    frequency as a test of the theory of the selective neu-
    trality of polymorphisms. *Genetics* 74:175-195.
MACCLUER, J. W. 1967. Montecarlo methods in human popula-
    tion genetics; a computer model incorporating age spe-
    cific birth and death rates. *Amer. J. Hum. Genet.* 19:
    303-312.
MALCOLM, L. A., P. B. BOOTH and L. L. CAVALLI-SFORZA. 1971.
    Intermarriage patterns and blood group gene frequencies
    of the Bundi people of the New Guinea Highlands. *Human
    Biology* 43:187-199.
MALECOT, G. 1950. Quelques schemas probabilistes sur la
    variabilite des populations naturelles. *Ann. Univ.
    Lyon Sci., A.* 13:37-60.
ROBERTS, D. F. and R. W. HIORNS. 1962. The dynamics of rac-
    ial intermixture. *Amer. J. Hum. Genet.* 14:261-277.
ROBERTSON, A. 1951. The analysis of heterogeneity in the
    binomial distribution. *Ann. Eugen.* 16:1-15.
SMITH, C. A. B. 1969. Local fluctuations in gene frequencies.
    Ann. Hum. Genet. 32:251-260.
WARD, R. and J. NEEL. 1970. Gene frequencies and microdif-
    ferentiation among the Makiritare Indians. IV. Compar-
    ison of a genetic network with ethnohistory and migration

matrices; a new index of genetic isolation. *Amer. J. Hum. Genet.* 22:538-561.

WRIGHT, S. 1943. Isolation by distance. *Genetics* 28: 114-138.

WRIGHT, S. 1931. Evolution in Mendelian populations. *Genetics* 6:144-161.

A NEW MEASURE OF GENETIC DISTANCE

Masatoshi Nei

*Division of Biological and Medical Sciences
Brown University, Providence, Rhode Island*

In recent years, several authors have proposed different measures of genetic distance between populations (CAVALLI-SFORZA and EDWARDS 1967, BALAKRISHNAN and SANGHVI 1969, HEDRICK 1971, and others). In many of them, however, it is not clear what biological unit they are going to measure. From the standpoint of genetics, the most appropriate measure of genetic distance would be the number of nucleotide or codon differences per unit length of DNA.

Theoretically, it is possible to determine the number of nucleotide differences by biochemical techniques. At the present time, however, sequencing of nucleotides is expensive and time-consuming even for a short length of DNA. DNA hybridization techniques now available are too crude to be used for detecting a small number of nucleotide differences that would occur among local populations within a species. Therefore, we are forced to use other methods. In view of this circumstance, I have proposed a statistical method by which the number of codon differences per locus can be estimated from gene frequency data (NEI 1971a, 1972). In this paper I shall discuss the outline of this method and some of the recent extensions. The results of the application of this method to some gene frequency data will also be discussed.

This work was supported in part by Public Health Service Grant GM-17719 and by National Science Foundation Grant GB-21224.

IDENTITY OF GENES AND GENETIC DISTANCE

Consider two populations, X and Y, in which multiple alleles are segregating at a locus. Let x_i and y_i be the frequencies of the ith alleles in X and Y, respectively. The probability of identity of two randomly chosen genes is $j_X = \Sigma x_i^2$ in population X, while it is $j_Y = \Sigma y_i^2$ in population Y. The probability of identity of a gene from X and a gene from Y is $j_{XY} = \Sigma x_i y_i$. If there is no selection and each allele is derived from a single mutation in an ancestral generation, the expected values of j_X and j_Y are equal to WRIGHT's coefficients of inbreeding in X and Y respectively, while that of j_{XY} is equal to MALECOT's (1967) coefficient of kinship. In the study of gene differences between populations, it is desirable to examine a large number of loci, which are ideally a random sample of the total genome, including both polymorphic and monomorphic loci.

We define the normalized identity of genes between X and Y as follows:

$$I = J_{XY}/\sqrt{J_X J_Y} \tag{1}$$

where J_X, J_Y and J_{XY} are the arithmetic means of j_X, j_Y and j_{XY} respectively, over all loci, including monomorphic loci. I is unity when the two populations have the same alleles with the same frequencies at all loci, while it is 0 when they have no common alleles at any locus. The genetic distance between X and Y is then measured by

$$D = -\log_e I \tag{2}$$

As will be seen later, this definition is quite appropriate if X and Y are sexually isolated and the rate of gene substitution per locus is the same for all loci. In this case, D measures the accumulated number of gene substitutions or codon differences per locus. Data on amino acid substitutions in some proteins, however, indicate that the rate of gene substitution varies considerably among loci (DAYHOFF 1969). If this rate is not the same for all loci, D gives an underestimate of the number of gene substitutions per locus (NEI 1971b).

When the rate of gene substitution varies with locus and all of I_j's are large, a more appropriate measure of genetic distance is given by

$$D' = -\log_e I' \tag{3}$$

where $I' = J'_{XY}/\sqrt{J'_X J'_Y}$, in which J'_X, J'_Y and J'_{XY} are the geometric means of j_X, j_Y and j_{XY}, respectively.

DIFFERENTIATION OF ISOLATED POPULATIONS

Suppose that a population splits into two isolated populations and thereafter no migration occurs between the two populations. Let I_0 be the normalized identity of genes between the two populations at the time of completion of sexual isolation. For simplicity, we assume that the effective sizes of the two populations are equal (N) and they are in a steady state in the sense that the effects of mutation, selection and genetic random drift are balanced. We further assume that each new mutation is an allele not pre-existing in any of the two populations. The probability of nucleotide substitution per DNA base per year or per generation is so small, that this assumption seems to be valid in most cases. Under these conditions, the value of j_X at a particular locus varies from time to time, but its expectation remains constant. When gene substitution occurs through neutral mutations, $E(j_X)$ is equal to $1/(4Nu + 1)$, where u is the rate of neutral mutations per generation (KIMURA and CROW 1964). If selection is important, $E(j_X)$ takes a more complicated form (cf. KIMURA 1969). At any rate, if a large number of loci are examined, J_X can be assumed to be constant and equal to $E(j_X)$. The same is true for J_Y. It is interesting to note that the average heterozygosity $(1 - J_X)$ for protein loci is about 0.1 and nearly the same for all the seven different organisms so far studied (KIMURA and OHTA 1971).

On the other hand, the expectation of j_{XY} gradually decreases as time goes on. Let α be the rate of gene substitution per locus per year. If neutral gene substitution is important, α is equal to the rate of neutral mutations per locus per year (KIMURA 1968, NEI 1969, CROW 1969, KING and JUKES 1969). If selection is important, it is given by $4Nsu'$, approximately, where s is the average selective advantage of a new mutation over the original allele and u' is the mutation rate per locus per year (KIMURA and OHTA 1971). If the rate of gene substitution varies with time, we can use the average value for α in the following formulation.

The expectation of the normalized identity of genes in the tth year after sexual isolation is then given by

$$E(j_{XY}^{(t)})[E(j_X^{(t)})E(j_Y^{(t)})]^{-1/2} = \frac{E(j_{XY}^{(0)})}{\sqrt{E(j_X^{(0)})E(j_Y^{(0)})}} e^{-2\alpha t} \quad (4)$$

or

$$I = I_0 e^{-2\alpha t} \quad (5)$$

The genetic distance D therefore becomes

$$D = 2\alpha t - \log_e I_0 \quad (6)$$

The value of I_0 would be close to 1 in most cases, so that the second term in the above formula can generally be neglected. It is clear that D is essentially the same as that of NEI (1971b) and measures the accumulated number of codon differences per locus between the two populations. Under certain circumstances, I_0 can be estimated (NEI 1972).

As mentioned earlier, when α varies with locus, D' may be a better estimate of the number of gene differences than D. Since the natural logarithm of

$$E(j_{XY}^{(t)})[E(j_X^{(t)})E(j_Y^{(t)})]^{-1/2}$$

at the jth locus is given by $-2\alpha_j t$, where α_j is the value of α at this locus and I_0 is assumed to be 1, D' can be written as

$$D' = 2(\alpha_1 + \alpha_2 + \ldots + \alpha_n)t/n$$

$$= 2\alpha_m t \quad (7)$$

where α_m is the average value of α_j. In practice, however, this value is affected by sampling errors of gene frequencies at the time of population survey as well as by genetic random drift to a considerable extent. These factors are expected generally to inflate the estimate of $2\alpha_m t$. If one of the I_j (the value of $j_{XY}/\sqrt{j_X j_Y}$ at the jth locus) is 0, D' becomes ∞.

The effect of these factors, however, would not be large if sample size is large and all of I_j's are larger than 0.7. At any rate, the true value of $2\alpha_m t$ is expected to be somewhere between D and D'.

GENETIC DISTANCE BETWEEN INCOMPLETELY ISOLATED POPULATIONS

If migration occurs between two populations, these populations always share some common alleles and the differentiation of the populations will be hindered. The steady-state relation between the identity of genes and migration rate can be worked out with certain population models. In this section we assume that there is no selection.

Island Model

MARUYAMA (1970) worked out the steady-state formulae for the expected values of j_X and j_{XY} in the island model with a finite number of subpopulations. Let N, n, m, and u be the size of a subpopulation, number of subpopulations, migration rate, and mutation rate per generation, respectively. Using MARUYAMA's results, it can be shown that, if $u \ll m$,

$$I = \frac{m(2-m)}{m(2-m) + 2nu(1-m)^2} \tag{8}$$

approximately. It is of interest to see that I is independent of N. I is unity when $u = 0$ or when $m = 1$, as it should be. On the other hand, $I = 0$ when $n = \infty$. In reality, of course, n is always finite.

From (8), we obtain

$$D = \log_e(1 + \frac{nu(1-m)^2}{m(1-m/2)}) \tag{9}$$

which becomes

$$D = \frac{nu(1-m)^2}{m(1-m/2)} \tag{10}$$

approximately, if $nu(1-m)^2/[m(1-m/2)]$ is smaller than 0.3. Most values of D between local populations appear to be much smaller than 0.3. Formula (10) indicates that D is linearly

related to the number of subpopulations. If the number of
subpopulations is linearly related to the geographical area
in which they are located, D becomes a linear function of
the area.

Steppingstone Model

With a linear steppingstone model (KIMURA and WEISS
1964), it can be shown that the normalized identity of genes
between subpopulations which are k steps apart is

$$I(k) = e^{-\sqrt{2u/m}\, k} \tag{11}$$

where m is the migration rate such that every generation a
proportion, m/2, of the genes in a population is exchanged
with its two neighboring subpopulations. The above formula
is correct only when the number of subpopulations is large.
Therefore, the genetic distance between two populations which
are k steps apart is given by

$$D(k) = \sqrt{2u/m}\, k \tag{12}$$

Thus, D(k) is linearly related to the geographical distance.

When the geographical distribution of individuals is
continuous rather than of the steppingstone type, (11) and
(12) also hold true if we replace m by σ^2, where σ^2 is the
variance of migration distance in a generation (MALECOT 1959).
With a two-dimensional steppingstone model or continuous distribution model, a similar formula can be derived, but in
this case D(x) is no longer linear with distance (MALECOT
1959, NEI 1972).

MALECOT (1959, 1967) has derived the following formula
for the relationship between coefficient of kinship (ϕ) and
distance (k).

$$\phi = ae^{-bk}/k^c$$

where a, b and c are constants. For a one-dimensional distribution, c = 0; for a two-dimensional distribution, c = 1/2.
This formula has been used by MORTON and his associates
(MORTON 1969) to study the genetic differentiation of human
populations. They have used gene frequency data for a single

polymorphic locus in fitting the above formula. Care should
be exercised, however, when the formula is to be applied to
a single-locus data. We know that about 30 percent of the
loci of the human genome are polymorphic (HARRIS 1969). It
is likely that a majority of these polymorphisms are tran -
sient, whether they are neutral or not. Therefore, at a
particular evolutionary time one locus may be polymorphic,
but at another time it may be monomorphic.

If MALECOT's formula is applied to a transient polymorphic locus, the meanings of the estimates of a and b are no
longer the same as the interpretations given by MALECOT. In
fact, the values of a and b vary from time to time or from
locus to locus even in the same population. This is especially so in relatively small populations. If the total population size is small, the distribution of gene frequency among
subpopulations varies considerably from time to time and even
a gene frequency cline for a neutral locus may arise (KIMURA
and MARUYAMA 1971). In these circumstances, positive values
of the estimates of a and b simply mean that the distance of
gene dispersal per generation is small compared with the total
area in which individuals are distributed. MORTON (1969, p.
65) is apparently aware of this difficulty, but he still
thinks that the comparison of estimates of a and b among
different populations is useful.

This difficulty is removed at least theoretically if we
use a large number of loci instead of a single locus, including monomorphic loci. In this case the normalized identity of
genes is given by (11) or the equivalent formula for a two-
dimensional distribution, if there is no selection. Therefore,
it is possible to estimate the value of $b = \sqrt{2u/m}$. If there
is selection, however, we do not know the exact relationship
between the normalized identity of genes and distance.

MINIMUM NUMBER OF CODON DIFFERENCES

In the foregoing sections we assumed that the populations
in question are in a steady state, so that the effects of
mutation, selection, migration, and genetic random drift are
balanced. In an arbitrary pair of popuations, however, this
assumption does not necessarily hold, so that the estimates
obtained by the present method may be incorrect. Fortunately,
it is possible to estimate a minimum number of codon differences between any pair of populations. Furthermore, the

estimate of minimum codon differences can be obtained even
between two randomly chosen genomes from the same population.

As was already shown, the probability of identity of two
genes drawn at random at a locus, one from each of populations X and Y, is j_{XY}. The probability that the two genes are
not the same is, therefore, $d_{XY} = 1 - j_{XY}$. At the nucleotide level, there must be at least one codon difference between any pair of different alleles (nucleotide sequences).
Thus, d_{XY} is a minimum estimate of the number of codon differences at this locus, while $D_{XY} = 1 - J_{XY}$ is a minimum
estimate of the average number of codon differences between
two randomly chosen genomes in X and Y, respectively. Therefore, $D_m = D_{XY} - (D_X + D_Y)/2$ is a *minimum estimate* of codon
differences between X and Y when the intrapopulational codon
differences are subtracted. D_m can also be computed as the
mean of $d = \Sigma(x_i - y_i)^2/2$ over all loci. Note that if X and
Y are randomly mating diploid populations, D_X and D_Y are
equal to the average heterozygosities in X and Y, respectively.

The value of D_m is always smaller than the estimate
obtained by formula (2) or (3). On the other hand, $D' =
-\log_e I'$ in (3) is always largest among the three estimates.
We will call this the *maximum estimate* of codon differences
between X and Y. Both minimum and maximum estimates refer,
of course, to those codon differences that are detectable by
the technique available (e.g. electrophoresis). Ordinarily,
there is not much difference between the three estimates when
applied to different races in the same species.

It is often interesting to know the interpopulational
codon differences relative to the intrapopulational differences. This ratio can be estimated by

$$R = 2D_m/(D_X + D_Y) \tag{13}$$

This value would not be affected appreciably by the detect-
ability of gene differences by a particular technique such
as electrophoresis, since both the numerator and denominator
will be affected equally.

CORRECTION FOR THE EFFECT OF INTERRACIAL MIXTURE

In recent years, there has been considerable interracial
mixing in man. For example, about 20 percent of American

Negro genes are believed to be of Caucasian origin, while virtually no Negro genes have entered the Caucasian gene pool (REED 1969). In these cases, it is possible to estimate the number of codon differences between two populations before interracial mixture occurred, if the proportions of foreign genes in the two populations are known.

We assume that interracial mixture occurred only recently, so that natural selection after gene mixture is negligible. We also assume that the population size is so large, that the effect of genetic random drift is unimportant. Let p be the proportion of genes in population X that comes from population Y, and q the proportion of genes in Y that comes from X. The expected identity of two randomly chosen genes in X is then given by

$$J_X = (1-p)^2 J_{X0} + 2p(1-p)J_{XY0} + p^2 J_{Y0}$$

where J_{X0}, J_{XY0} and J_{Y0} are the identity of genes corresponding to J_X, J_{XY} and J_Y, respectively, before interracial mixture occurred. Similarly,

$$J_{XY} = (1-p)qJ_{X0} + (1-p-q+2pq)J_{XY0} + p(1-q)J_{Y0}$$

$$J_Y = q^2 J_X + 2q(1-q)J_{XY} + (1-q)^2 J_Y$$

Therefore, the values of J_{X0}, J_{XY0} and J_{Y0} can be estimated by the following formula. (14)

$$
\begin{pmatrix} J_{X0} \\ J_{XY0} \\ J_{Y0} \end{pmatrix}
= (1-p-q)^{-2}
\begin{pmatrix}
(1-q)^2 & -2p(1-q) & p^2 \\
-q(1-q) & (1-p-q+2pq) & -p(1-p) \\
q^2 & 2(1-p)q & (1-p)^2
\end{pmatrix}
\begin{pmatrix} J_X \\ J_{XY} \\ J_Y \end{pmatrix}
$$

This formula has been applied to estimate the genetic distance between Caucasians and African Negroes from data on Caucasians and American Negroes (NEI and ROYCHOUDHURY 1974).

SOME NUMERICAL EXAMPLES

In order to know interpopulational gene differences
within a species, we have applied our method to gene frequency data for *Drosophila pseudoobscura*, the house mouse
and man. The results for *D. pseudoobscura* are presented in
TABLE I. The data used for this study were obtained by
PRAKASH et al. (1969). They studied the gene frequencies
for 24 protein loci in three United States populations
(Strawberry Canyon, California; Mesa Verde, Colorado; Austin,
Texas) and one Colombian (Bogota) population. The estimates
of D in TABLE I were obtained by using (2). It is seen that
the value of D is rather small and less than 0.01 among the
three United States populations. The minimum estimates of
codon differences (D_m) among these populations are only
slightly smaller than those of D. The interpopulational
codon differences relative to the intrapopulational codon
differences (R) can be computed from the values of J_X and
J_{XY} in TABLE I. The average value of this ratio for the three
pairs of United States populations is 0.048. Thus, the interpopulational codon differences are only 5 percent of the
intrapopulational codon differences, which is equal to 0.12.

The Bogota population is considerably different from the
United States populations, as was already noted by PRAKASH
et al. (1969). The genetic distance between the populations
in the two countries is, on the average, more than 10 times
larger than that between the United States populations.
Particularly, the distance (0.126) between the Bogota and
Austin populations is close to the distance between semispecies in the house mouse (NEI 1972). The average value of
minimum estimates of codon differences between the Bogota and
other populations is 0.096, while the intrapopulational codon
differences in the Bogota population is 0.045. Thus, the
former is twice as large as the latter. The reason for the
relatively small amount of genetic variability in the Bogota
population has been discussed by PRAKASH et al. (1969).

In the house mouse, the numbers of codon differences
between two semispecies *(Mus musculus musculus* and *M. m.
domesticus)*, as well as between local populations in the same
semispecies were studied (NEI 1972). The gene frequency data
(41 protein loci) were those obtained by SELANDER et al.
(1969). The estimate of the number of codon differences detected by electrophoresis was 0.03 or less between local
populations, while it was 0.13 $\sim$ 0.20 between the two

TABLE I

ESTIMATES OF J_X, J_{XY} AND D FOR FOUR POPULATIONS

OF *DROSOPHILA MELANOGASTER*

	Strawberry Canyon	Mesa Verde	Austin	Bogota
Strawberry Canyon	(.8597)	.0078	.0098	.0827
Mesa Verde	.8680	(.8902)	.0026	.1219
Austin	.8629	.8844	(.8833)	.1260
Bogota	.8347	.8168	.8103	(.9564)

The values on the diagonal are J_X. The values above
the diagonal are D and the values below the diagonal
are J_{XY}. These values were computed from the data by
PRAKASH et al. (1969).

semispecies.

   The gene differences between Caucasian and Negro populations in man is also rather small compared with those within
the same population (NEI and ROYCHOUDHURY unpublished). The
minimum number of interpopulational codon differences, estimated from 44 protein loci, was 0.01, while the minimum
estimate of intrapopulational codon differences were 0.10.
Therefore, the former is only 10 percent of the latter.
These results suggest that the genes in Caucasian and Negro
populations are remarkably similar, although the phenotypic
differences in such characters as pigmentation and facial
structures are conspicuous. It is likely that the genes responsible for these characters were subjected to stronger
natural selection than "average genes" in the process of
racial differentiation.

   From the results mentioned above for the three different
species, it may be concluded that the number of electrophoretically detectable codon differences is roughly 0.1 or less
per locus between local populations of a species, while it is
larger than 0.1 between semispecies. The Bogota population

in *D. pseudoobscura* appears to be on the borderline between local race and semispecies when compared with the United States populations. NEI (1971b) studied electrophoretically detectable gene differences between different species of *Drosophila*. The average value of D for a pair of sibling species was 0.76, while it was 1.86 for a pair of nonsibling species. LAKOVAARA et al. (1972) obtained similar values for a different group of Drosophila. Of course, the number of populations or species so far studied is very small, so that our tentative figures may be revised considerably in the future. Furthermore, the definition of species or semi-species depends on reproductive isolation as well as on genic or morphological differences. Therefore, it is not surprising to find many exceptions to the general rule mentioned above.

As noted by NEI (1971b), the present method does not give reliable estimates when I is close to 0. However, if substitution of synonymous codons is disregarded, $2\alpha t$ can be written as $2n\lambda t$, where n is the number of amino acids that compose a polypeptide and λ is the average rate of amino acid substitution per residue per year. Therefore, if amino acid sequence data are available, the value of D can be estimated even for a pair of distantly related species. Of course, this value of D cannot be directly compared with the D estimated from electrophoretic data on protein identity, since electro-phoresis detects only a portion of amino acid differences. See NEI (1971b) for a detailed discussion of this problem.

As an example, let us consider the genetic distance be-tween man and horse. It is known that the number of amino acid differences between β chains of human and horse hemo-globin is 25. Since a β chain polypeptide consists of 146 amino acids, $2\lambda t$ can be estimated by $-\log_e(1-25/146)$, which becomes 0.188. Multiplying this number by n = 146, we get $2n\lambda t$ = 27.4 for the β chain. However, hemoglobin β chain is a relatively small polypeptide. The "average polypeptide" appears to consist of some 400 amino acids (NEI 1971b). Thus, the genetic distance between man and horse would be roughly 75 codon differences per locus. To get a more reliable esti-mate, of course, we must examine many different protein data.

SUMMARY

A measure of genetic distance based on the identity of genes between populations is discussed. This distance is

intended to measure the number of accumulated codon differences per locus between populations. Methods for obtaining
a minimum and a maximum estimate of this number are presented.
Some of the results of the application of these methods to
gene frequency data for *Drosophila pseudoobscura*, the house
mouse and man are discussed. It seems that the number of
electrophoretically detectable codon differences between
local populations of a species is less than 0.1 per locus
except for some unusual case.

LITERATURE CITED

BALAKRISHNAN, V. and L. D. SANGHVI. 1968. Distance between
    populations on the basis of attribute data. *Biometrics*
    24:859-865.
CAVALLI-SFORZA, L. L. and A. W. F. EDWARDS. 1967. Phylo-
    genetic analysis: models and estimation procedures.
    Amer. J. Human Genet. 19:233-257.
CROW, J. F. 1969. Molecular genetics and population genetics.
    Proc. XII Intern. Congr. Genet., Vol. 3, pp. 105-113.
DAYHOFF, M. O. 1969. *Atlas of Protein Sequence and Structure,
    1969*. National Biomedical Research Foundation, Washington
HARRIS, H. 1969. Enzyme and protein polymorphism in human
    populations. *British Med. Bull.* 25:5-13.
HEDRICK, P. W. 1971. A new approach to measuring genetic
    similarity. *Evolution* 25:276-280.
KIMURA, M. 1968. Evolutionary rate at the molecular level.
    Nature 217:624-626.
KIMURA, M. 1969. The number of heterozygous nucleotide
    sites maintained in a finite population due to steady
    flux of mutations. *Genetics* 61:893-903.
KIMURA, M. and J. F. CROW. 1964. The number of alleles that
    can be maintained in a finite population. *Genetics* 49:
    725-738.
KIMURA, M. and T. MARUYAMA. 1971. Pattern of neutral poly-
    morphism in a geographically structured population.
    Genet. Res. 18:125-131.
KIMURA, M. and T. OHTA. 1971. Protein polymorphism as a
    phase of molecular evolution. *Nature* 229:467-469.
KIMURA, M. and G. WEISS. 1964. The steppingstone model of
    population structure and the decrease of genetic cor-
    relation with distance. *Genetics* 49:561-567.
KING, J. L. and T. H. JUKES. 1969. Non-Darwinian evolution.
    Science 164:788-798.
LAKOVAARA, S., A. SAURA and C. T. FALLS. 1972. Genetic

distance and evolutionary relationships in the *Drosophila obscura* group. *Evolution* 26:177-184.

MALECOT, G. 1959. Les modeles stochastiques en genetique de population. *Publ. Inst. Statist. Univ. Paris* 8:173-210.

MALECOT, G. 1967. Identical loci and relationship. *Proc. Vth Berkeley Symp. Math. Statist. Probabil.*, Vol. 4, pp. 317-332.

MARUYAMA, T. 1970. Effective number of alleles in a subdivided population. *Theoret. Popul. Biol.* 1:273-306.

MORTON, N. E. 1969. Human population structure. *Ann. Rev. Genet.* 3:53-74.

NEI, M. 1969. Gene duplication and nucleotide substitution in evolution. *Nature* 221:40-43.

NEI, M. 1971a. Identity of genes and genetic distance between populations. *Genetics* 68:s47.

NEI, M. 1971b. Interspecific gene differences and evolutionary time estimated from electrophoretic data on protein identity. *Amer. Nat.* 105:385-398.

NEI, M. 1972. Genetic distance between populations. *Amer. Nat.* 106:283-292.

NEI, M. and A. K. ROYCHOUDHURY. 1972. Gene differences between Caucasian, Negro, and Japanese populations. *Science* 177:434-436.

NEI, M. and A. K. ROYCHOUDHURY. 1974. Genic variation within and between the three major races of man, Caucasoids, Negroids, and Mongoloids. *Amer. J. Hum. Genet.* 26 (in press).

PRAKASH, S., R. C. LEWONTIN and J. L. HUBBY. 1969. A molecular approach to the study of genic heterozygosity in natural populations. IV. Patterns of genic variation in central, marginal and isolated populations of *Drosophila pseudoobscura*. *Genetics* 61:841-858.

REED, T. E. 1969. Caucasian genes in American Negroes. *Science* 165:841-858.

SELANDER, R. K., W. G. HUNT and S. Y. YANG. 1969. Protein polymorphism and genic heterozygosity in two European subspecies of the house mouse. *Evolution* 23:279-390.

MONTE CARLO SIMULATION: THE EFFECTS OF MIGRATION ON SOME MEASURES OF GENETIC DISTANCE

Jean W. MacCluer

Departments of Biology and Anthropology
The Pennsylvania State University
University Park, Pennsylvania

Genetic distances, and the genetic networks derived from them, have been used to reconstruct probable relationships among human populations and to trace their descent from some common ancestral group. But, if gene frequency data are to be used as a means of deducing the relatedness of populations, then one needs information on the effects of mating practices, nonrandom migration, and age-dependent fertility and mortality on genetic differentiation. For most human populations which are suitable for genetic study, the necessary data on population history, in particular on population numbers and on rates of birth, death, and migration through time, are unavailable. Equally troublesome is the inadequacy of data on genetic differences in fertility, mortality, and nuptiality, and the uncertainty as to the possible influence of such selection on genetic differentiation. In short, very little is known about the expected behavior of genetic distances under various genetic and demographic conditions. We would seem to be in the awkward position of trying to investigate the factors which influence distance measures by studying human populations, and also trying to study the relatedness of these populations by computing distance measures.

This work has been supported by grant GS-27382 of the National Science Foundation. Work on the computer model was begun at the Department of Human Genetics, The University of Michigan, and was supported there by grant AT(11-1)-1552 of the U. S. Atomic Energy Commission.

Perhaps the most valuable contribution of Monte Carlo simulation to studies of genetic distance will be in providing standards against which the behavior of populations can be judged. By creating computer models of populations and simulating their various demographic and genetic characteristics, one can maintain careful control over factors such as birth, death, and migration rates and selection coefficients, and observe the effects of various combinations of these on genetic differentiation. Only when it is known how certain types of populations may be expected to differentiate, for example, in the absence of selection and under constant random migration, will it be possible to evaluate the distances and resulting genetic networks derived for actual human populations.

As part of a larger project designed to investigate the relationship between demographic and genetic characteristics of human populations, we have begun to do computer simulations of some model human populations, all subjected to the same fertility and mortality schedules but undergoing different *controlled* amounts of migration between subpopulations. Our initial efforts have been directed to two problems, each of which will be discussed briefly: (1) determining some of the effects of migration on various measures of genetic differentiation for loci which are not subjected to selection, and whose alleles are at intermediate frequencies, and (2) investigating the genotype distributions in age-structured subdivided populations at various migration levels. The measures which were used in this study are arc distance (BHATTACHARYYA 1946), chord distance (CAVALLI-SFORZA and EDWARDS 1967), F_{ST} (WRIGHT 1943, 1951), and the related quantities F_{IS} and F_{IT} (WRIGHT 1943, 1951). The definitions of these measures are given in the Appendix.

THE SIMULATIONS

The simulation model used here, which was written for the IBM 360/67 computer, is a modification of models which have been described elsewhere (MacCLUER 1967, MacCLUER and SCHULL 1970, MacCLUER et al. 1971). The simulations were begun with an initial model population of size 400, divided into four villages each consisting of 50 males and 50 females, and all having identical age-sex structures and family compositions. Individuals were allowed to marry, reproduce, migrate, and die according to constant age- and sex-specific probabilities. The age-sex structure of the initial population and the probabilities of dying were taken from *Regional Model Life Tables and Stable Populations* (COALE and DEMENY 1966). A high rate of mortality (level seven east) was chosen, with an expected annual rate of increase of .5 percent. This slight positive rate of increase assured that the artificial populations would not die out during the course of the simulations. The fertility schedule was derived from a United Nations model age pattern of fertility (1965), the pattern chosen being a high-fertility, broad-peak type compiled from data from thirteen countries. The model population had a mean expectation of life at birth of 35.0 for females and 32.0 for males, mean generation times of 29.0 for females and 32.5 for males, and crude birth rates of 33.2 for females and 35.9 for males.

Ten computer runs were done, each beginning with the same model population of 400 individuals, and each simulating 200 years of the population's vital events, thus generating ten artificial pedigrees. Some demographic characteristics of the ten populations are given in TABLE I. It can be seen that, although the populations have experienced different rates of migration between villages, there are no systematic differences in their other demographic characteristics.

TABLE   I

SOME DEMOGRAPHIC CHARACTERISTICS OF TEN ARTIFICIAL POPULATIONS

RUN	MIGRA-TION RATE	POPULATION SIZE (YEAR 200)	BIRTHS	DEATHS	MAR-RIAGES	MIGRA-TIONS
1	0	648	3549	3301	1184	0
2	0	824	4216	3792	1441	0
3	0	847	4251	3804	1352	0
4	.00125	778	4274	3896	1395	143
5	.00125	895	4509	4014	1458	156
6	.0025	779	3977	3598	1310	223
7	.0025	848	4100	3652	1335	290
8	.005	827	3799	3372	1228	483
9	.01	587	3249	3062	1034	870
10	.01	630	3539	3309	1152	934

TABLE   I   (cont.)

RUN	AGE AT PATERNITY		AGE AT MATERNITY		BIRTH INTERVAL		COMPLETED LIVEBIRTHS		FAMILY SIZE SURVIVING OFFSPRING	
	μ	σ^2	μ	σ^2	μ	σ^2	μ	σ^2	μ	σ^2
1	33.0	99.7	29.1	54.3	4.22	11.8	4.22	3.88	2.45	2.52
2	32.0	93.0	28.8	54.1	4.28	12.2	4.37	3.87	2.50	2.39
3	32.5	95.2	29.0	54.4	4.17	11.6	4.50	3.89	2.57	2.44
4	32.2	93.1	28.7	55.2	4.29	12.3	4.31	3.83	2.57	2.52
5	32.5	94.0	28.8	55.1	4.32	12.6	4.35	3.73	2.61	2.37
6	32.1	94.8	29.0	56.9	4.35	12.8	4.18	4.27	2.62	3.20
7	32.1	93.1	29.0	54.3	4.19	11.6	4.41	3.73	2.67	2.68
8	32.4	94.5	28.9	55.7	4.28	12.1	4.45	4.22	2.77	2.84
9	32.4	94.1	28.9	54.5	4.35	13.4	4.33	3.44	2.81	2.70
10	32.3	87.9	29.0	54.9	4.42	12.8	4.01	4.11	2.71	2.92
MEAN	32.4	93.9	28.9	54.9	4.29	12.3	4.31	3.90	2.63	2.66

For each of the ten pedigrees, gene segregation was
simulated for 60 biallelic loci, all at an initial frequency
of .50. In the initial population, genotypes of adults (age
15 and over) were assigned randomly, with genotype frequencies
for each locus held at Hardy-Weinberg equilibrium within each
village. Genotypes for children in the initial population
(i.e. all individuals under age 15) were assigned so as to be
consistent with those of their parents, and were also in
Hardy-Weinberg frequencies. Descendants of the initial population were assigned genotypes on the basis of the genotypes
of their parents.

THE EFFECT OF MIGRATION ON F_{ST} AND GENETIC DISTANCES

After all individuals in a pedigree had been assigned
genotypes for each of the 60 loci, several measures of genetic
distance were computed. The calculations were done for all
60 loci and, as a basis for comparison with typical data from
actual human populations, for three sets of 20 loci each and
six sets of 10 loci each. Because all the villages initially
had identical Hardy-Weinberg distributions of genotypes, all
the distances were zero at the beginning of each simulation
run.

Our first objective was to impose varying amounts of
migration on the artificial populations and to determine how

much migration was necessary to produce a noticeable reduction
in the amount of genetic differentiation between villages, as
compared with isolated villages. In the simulations, single
adults were allowed to migrate alone, married men took with
them their wives and children, and widowed adults took their
children. Migrants from each village were equally likely to
go to any of the other three villages, but there was no out-
migration. For this study, migration probabilities were constant across all ages. Initially, three pedigrees were
generated in which there was no migration between villages.
For the next two runs, the yearly migration rate was set at
.01; it was successively halved in subsequent runs until it
was judged that the various measures of genetic differentiation were not significantly different from those of the three
populations of isolated villages. We found excellent agreement between the probabilities of migration specified as
input, and the observed migration rates as calculated from
each of the resulting artificial pedigrees, thus giving us
confidence that we were able to control the rate of migration
well.

TABLE II shows values of F_{ST} at the end of 200 years,
averaged across all 60 loci, for the ten runs at various
migration levels. As would be expected, F_{ST} decreases with
increasing exchange between villages. F_{ST} values for populations at migration level .01 are quite different from those
for populations with no migration; there is no detectable
difference, however, between F_{ST}'s for runs with no migration and with rate .00125. It should be recalled that these
are *yearly*, not generational, migration rates, with the runs
having between 143 and 934 migrants in 200 years. As indicated in TABLE II, a yearly rate of .00125, for example,
corresponds to a rate of about 3.75 percent per generation.
F_{ST} was computed in two ways, from σ^2/pq and from $(F_{IT} -
F_{IS})/(1 - F_{IS})$, the results of the two calculations usually
differing only in the fourth decimal place. The agreement
between the two values, which is excellent even when the
analysis is based on only ten loci, may be taken as an indication of random differentiation of subpopulations. As a
rule, F_{IT} and F_{IS} have been computed in this paper by CANNINGS
and EDWARDS' (1969) formula, which corrects for the effects
of small population size. However, it can be shown that the
relationship $F_{ST} = (F_{IT} - F_{IS})/(1 - F_{IS})$ does not hold if
the corrected F_{IT} and F_{IS} are used. Therefore, uncorrected
values have been used to calculate the F_{ST} values in the last
column of TABLE II.

TABLE II

F_{ST} AFTER 200 YEARS, FOR POPULATIONS WITH

DIFFERENT YEARLY MIGRATION RATES BETWEEN SUBDIVISIONS

MIGRATION RATE		NO. OF	POPULATION		
PER YEAR	PER GENERATION	MIGRANTS IN 200 YRS	SIZE IN YEAR 200	F_{ST} *	F_{ST} **
0	0	0	648	.0300	.0303
0	0	0	824	.0275	.0276
0	0	0	847	.0212	.0207
.00125	.0375	143	778	.0229	.0233
.00125	.0375	156	895	.0267	.0266
.0025	.075	223	779	.0171	.0171
.0025	.075	290	848	.0201	.0202
.005	.150	483	827	.0175	.0176
.01	.300	870	587	.0111	.0109
.01	.300	934	630	.0115	.0116

$$*F_{ST} = \sigma_q^2 / \overline{pq}$$

$$**F_{ST} = (F_{IT} - F_{IS})/(1 - F_{IS})$$

If, as suggested by WORKMAN and NISWANDER (1970), it can be assumed that $2NF_{ST} = \chi^2$, where N is population size, then the significance of the differences between these values of F_{ST} can be tested by forming a ratio of χ^2's, which follows an F distribution. F ratios were computed, comparing F_{ST}'s for each run in which there was no migration with F_{ST}'s for runs at the various migration levels. Comparisons were also made between runs with migration level .00125 and runs with higher yearly migration rates. The significance of the differences between the various pairs of F_{ST}'s is indicated by the p values listed in TABLE III. The runs shown in each column, in which the yearly migration rate is 0 or .00125, appear in the numerators of the F ratios, and the runs listed in each row form the denominators. It should be noted that

TABLE III

P VALUES FOR COMPARISONS OF F_{ST} (AVERAGED OVER 60 LOCI)

IN ARTIFICIAL POPULATIONS AT DIFFERENT YEARLY MIGRATION RATES

MIGRATION RATE		0			.00125	
	RUN	1	2	3	4	5
0	2	.10-.25				
	3	.50-.75	.95			
.00125	4	.50-.75	.90-.95	.50-.75		
	5	.10	.25-.50	.05	.05	
.0025	6	.995	>.999	.975-.999	.975	>.999
	7	.75-.90	.975	.50-.75	.50-.75	.990
.005	8	.975	.999	.90-.95	.90-.95	.995-.999
.01	9	≫.999	≫.999	≫.999	≫.999	≫.999
	10	≫.999	≫.999	≫.999	≫.999	≫.999

$$F(180,180) = \frac{2N_{T_1} F_{ST_1}}{2N_{t_2} F_{ST_2}}$$

since the figure in the denominator of the F ratio always refers to a population with a migration rate as high or higher
than that in the numerator, one would expect the F ratio to
be greater than or equal to one, so that it would seem valid
to perform one-sided tests. Thus, p values of .99 would indicate significant differences between populations in the
expected direction, whereas p values of .01 would indicate
significant differences in the opposite direction. It can be
seen that, in general, the significance of the differences in
F_{ST} between runs tends to increase within each column as the
rate of migration increases, with consistently high levels of
significance at yearly migration rates of .005 and above. No
clear difference in F_{ST} is apparent, however, between runs
with no migration and those with a yearly rate of .125 percent.

Arc and chord distances were also computed for each of
the ten runs. TABLE IV shows arc distances between pairs of

TABLE   IV

ARC DISTANCES AFTER 200 YEARS (AVERAGED OVER 60 LOCI),
FOR POPULATIONS WITH
DIFFERENT YEARLY MIGRATION RATES BETWEEN SUBDIVISIONS

PAIRWISE DISTANCES

YEARLY MIGRATION RATE	1 - 2	1 - 3	1 - 4	2 - 3	2 - 4	3 - 4
0	.083	.060	.084	.069	.081	.086
0	.082	.072	.064	.069	.073	.070
0	.067	.061	.060	.075	.073	.066
.00125	.059	.075	.066	.059	.061	.071
.00125	.070	.058	.079	.067	.074	.069
.0025	.052	.057	.051	.063	.045	.055
.0025	.055	.070	.060	.062	.051	.060
.005	.056	.065	.065	.058	.046	.052
.01	.040	.039	.044	.053	.041	.052
.01	.051	.037	.042	.044	.051	.041

villages, averaged over 60 loci, for each migration level.
Again, populations with no migration are not readily dis-
tinguishable, on the basis of the arc distances between villages, from populations undergoing migration at the rate of
.125 percent per year; whereas, migration at yearly rates of
.5 percent and above is readily detected. An examination of
the corresponding chord distances for these runs led to the
same conclusion. Thus, at least over a 200 year period,
neither genetic distances nor F_{ST}'s are noticeably affected
even by migration rates as high as .125 percent per year, or
about 3.75 percent per generation.

Whereas the above analyses were done for 60 loci in each
pedigree, most studies of actual human populations include
between 10 and 20 loci. When the 60 loci for each run were
divided into six sets of 10 loci each, values of F_{ST} and pairwise distances between villages for each pedigree often dif-
fered by more than a factor of two, depending on which set of

TABLE V

PAIRWISE GENETIC DISTANCES AND F_{ST} FOR SIX SETS

OF TEN LOCI EACH, IN POPULATIONS WITH YEARLY

MIGRATION RATES OF 0, .00125 AND .0025

YEARLY MIGRA- TION RATE	RUN	SET	GENETIC DISTANCES						
			1-2	1-3	1-4	2-3	2-4	3-4	F_{ST}
0	3	1	.0729	.0573	.0567	.0795	.0640	.0539	.0170
		2	.0646	.0637	.0556	.0752	.0806	.0411	.0195
		3	.0844	.0579	.0531	.0936	.0877	.0740	.0217
		4	.0670	.0646	.0625	.0567	.0739	.0735	.0231
		5	.0510	.0550	.0638	.0550	.0606	.0582	.0181
		6	.0611	.0672	.0653	.0928	.0691	.0971	.0278
.00125	5	1	.0680	.0564	.0534	.0516	.0714	.0632	.0199
		2	.0700	.0712	.1152	.0803	.0799	.0668	.0337
		3	.0677	.0346	.0698	.0514	.0577	.0486	.0154
		4	.0699	.0587	.0825	.0766	.0839	.1109	.0339
		5	.0567	.0586	.0583	.0532	.0577	.0670	.0197
		6	.0863	.0715	.0927	.0914	.0958	.0551	.0376
.0025	6	1	.0761	.0705	.0559	.0623	.0410	.0535	.0196
		2	.0382	.0450	.0356	.0674	.0387	.0631	.0122
		3	.0336	.0568	.0397	.0517	.0391	.0776	.0122
		4	.0421	.0673	.0535	.0658	.0502	.0542	.0166
		5	.0419	.0389	.0453	.0590	.0664	.0235	.0159
		6	.0813	.0664	.0752	.0727	.0355	.0559	.0259

loci was used as the basis for the calculation. For example, TABLE V lists the values of F_{ST} and arc distance for six sets of 10 loci each for three pedigrees with yearly migration rates of 0, .00125 and .0025, respectively. If differences of this magnitude can arise even for selectively neutral loci at intermediate frequencies, then conclusions for real human populations, based on gene frequencies at 10 to 20 loci subjected to unknown selective pressures, must be considered tenuous at best.

TABLE VI

MEANS AND STANDARD DEVIATIONS FOR F_{IS}, F_{IT} AND F_{ST}

AFTER 200 YEARS (FOR 60 LOCI), FOR POPULATIONS WITH

DIFFERENT YEARLY MIGRATION RATES BETWEEN SUBDIVISIONS

YEARLY MIGRA-TION RATE	POPULATION SIZE IN YEAR 200	F_{IS}		F_{IT}		F_{ST}	
		μ	σ	μ	σ	μ	σ
0	648	−.0211	.0456	.0072	.0551	.0300	.0263
0	824	.0013	.0404	.0272	.0420	.0275	.0212
0	847	−.0025	.0487	.0165	.0504	.0212	.0178
.00125	778	−.0145	.0384	.0071	.0433	.0229	.0190
.00125	895	−.0139	.0430	.0102	.0465	.0267	.0206
.0025	779	−.0097	.0390	.0057	.0406	.0171	.0148
.0025	848	−.0075	.0405	.0111	.0397	.0201	.0165
.005	827	−.0060	.0398	.0100	.0388	.0175	.0132
.01	587	−.0073	.0500	.0011	.0505	.0111	.0093
.01	630	−.0017	.0477	.0074	.0501	.0115	.0099

DISTRIBUTIONS OF THE F STATISTICS

The various measures of genetic differentiation are a
function only of the sizes of the subpopulations and their
gene frequencies, and do not depend directly on the distribution of genes among the genotypes at each locus. However,
the genotype distributions are of interest as an indicator
of the rate at which drift is likely to occur, and therefore
of the rate of genetic differentiation between subpopulations.
In an effort to determine the extent to which age-structured
subdivided populations are likely to deviate from Hardy-
Weinberg genotype frequencies, we computed, for each of the
60 loci in each pedigree, WRIGHT's F_{IS} and F_{IT}, the former
measuring the average deviation of each subdivision from its
Hardy-Weinberg frequencies, and the latter measuring the
deviation of the entire population from Hardy-Weinberg
proportions. A summary of the means and standard deviations

for F_{IS} and F_{IT}, as well as F_{ST}, across all 60 loci for each of the ten pedigrees, is shown in TABLE VI. It can be seen that the mean value of F_{IS}, which was computed using the CANNINGS and EDWARDS (1969) correction for small population size, is nearly always negative. This pattern, which is observed fairly consistently throughout the 200 years of each run, can perhaps be accounted for by avoidance of close consanguinity, by slight differences in gene frequency between males and females (HALDANE 1954, WORKMAN 1969, CANNINGS and EDWARDS 1969) or by the variation in fertility in the population (PURSER 1966). Negative values of F_{IS} were also a consistent finding in experiments with another simulation model of a polygynous tribal population (NEEL & WARD, 1972). By continuing to simulate various types of model demographic structures, we hope to be able to determine how characteristic this phenomenon is of human populations.

The distributions of F_{IS}, F_{IT}, and F_{ST} through time, for one run in which there was no migration, are given in FIGURES 1, 2 and 3, respectively. It can be seen that the distributions of both F_{IS} and F_{IT} have large variances, even after only 50 years of differentiation, but that the variances do not change rapidly during the next 150 years. This study is being extended to larger numbers of loci, so that the shapes of the distributions can be determined more accurately. By computing the F statistics and their distributions for artificial populations under known demographic and genetic conditions, we hope to provide a standard of comparison for real human populations. It appears, however, that the variances of F_{IS} and F_{IT} are large enough that considerably more than ten to twenty loci will be required to obtain reliable estimates. Furthermore, it will be virtually impossible to detect the presence of selection by examining the F statistics for individual loci.

Finally, it is possible to look at the changes in distances and F statistics through time in the artificial populations. As an example, FIGURE 4 shows F_{IT} over a 200 year period in a run with yearly migration rate .01. Each of the three curves shows average F_{IT} computed for one set of 20 loci. It is interesting to note (1) the considerable variation from one set of 20 loci to the next within this pedigree, and (2) the large fluctuations through time for each set of loci. If such temporal fluctuations exist in real populations, then it will be difficult to draw general conclusions about population structure on the basis of F statistics com-

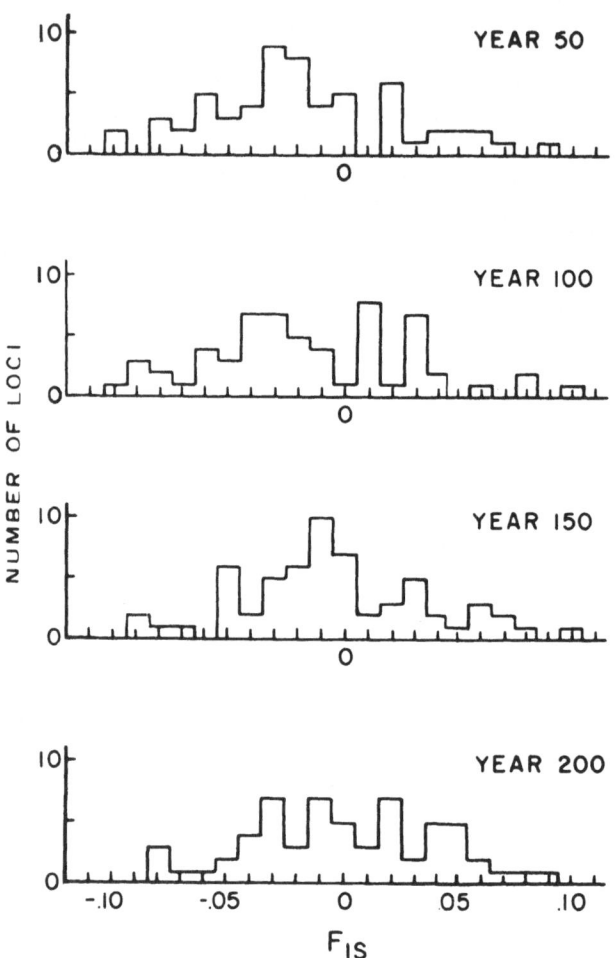

FIGURE 1.   Distribution of F_{IS} for 60 loci in an artificial population with no migration between subdivisions.

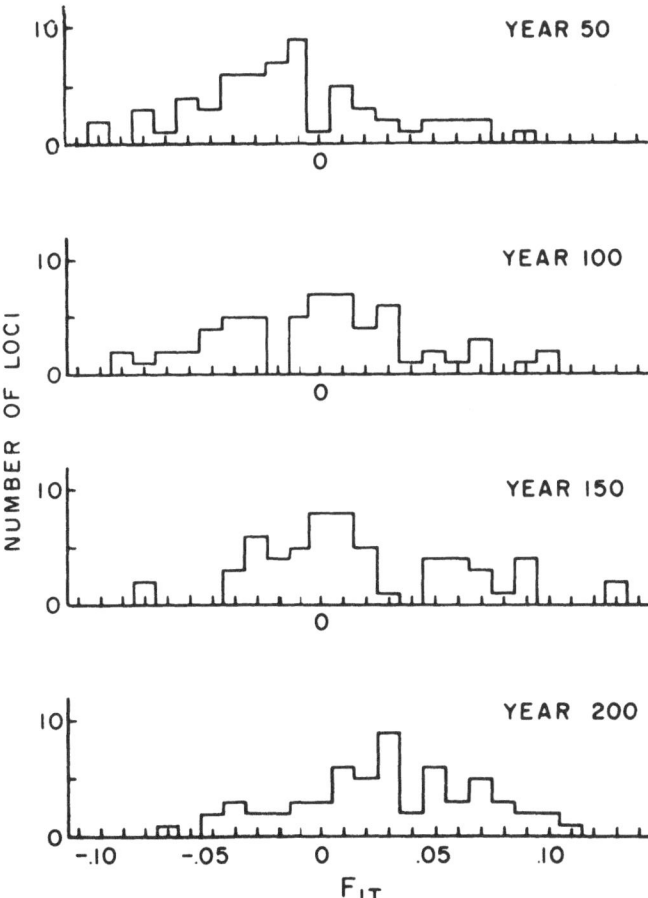

FIGURE 2.   Distribution of F_{IT} for 60 loci in an artificial
population with no migration between subdivisions.

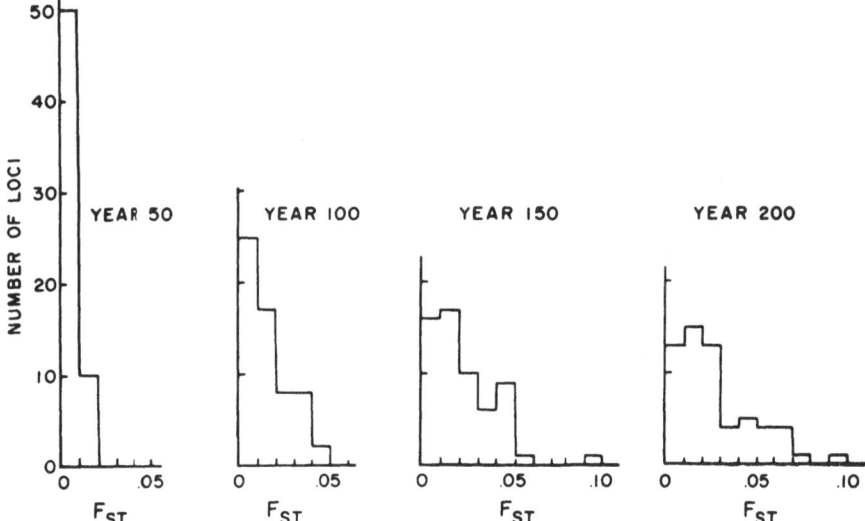

FIGURE 3. Distribution of F_{ST} for 60 loci in an artificial population with no migration between subdivisions.

puted at a single point in time. On the other hand, if it could be shown that F statistics in real populations are more stable through time, then we might have reason to believe that systematic pressures are responsible.

CONCLUSION

In cases where existing theory is inadequate, it is often possible to derive expected values and distributions of genetic parameters from computer simulation experiments. As an illustration of this use of Monte Carlo simulation, we have discussed two problems concerning the distributions of genes and genotypes in subdivided populations: (1) determining the effects of migration between subpopulations on three measures of genetic differentiation: arc distance, chord distance, and F_{ST}; and, (2) examining the distributions of the F statistics and their variability through time. Our preliminary findings are that:

1. As expected, genetic differentiation is greatest when villages are isolated from each other; however, even

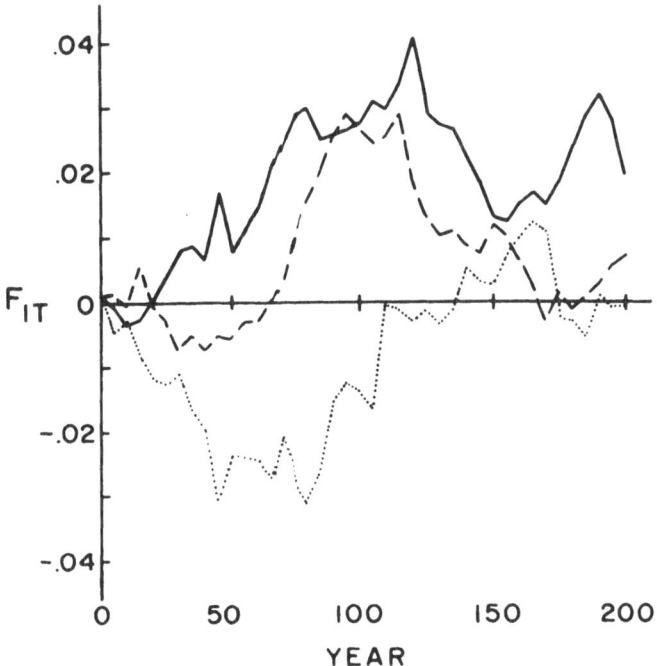

FIGURE 4. F_{IT} through time for 3 sets of 20 loci in an artificial population with yearly migration rate .01

when villages are exchanging migrants at a rate as high as 3.75 percent per generation for 200 years, genetic differentiation between villages is not noticeably diminished;

2. When pairwise genetic distances and F_{ST}'s are calculated for a pedigree from several sets of ten or twenty loci each, the results are quite variable, even though all loci begin at a frequency of .50 and all are selectively neutral;

3. F_{ST}'s calculated from $\sigma_q^2/\overline{pq}$ and $(F_{IT}-F_{IS})/(1-F_{IS})$ are nearly identical, as would be expected for randomly differentiating subpopulations;

4. Mean F_{IS} is consistently negative in these experiments;

5. The distributions of F_{IS} and F_{IT} have large variances; and

6. The temporal variability in F_{IS} and F_{IT} (and, to some extent, in F_{ST}) is rather large.

We are using Monte Carlo simulation to investigate gene and genotype distributions in subdivided populations at different fertility and mortality levels, for a range of initial gene frequencies, and for various patterns and intensities of selection. It will be of interest to do similar analyses in artificial populations which are interbreeding freely, and in those with progressively greater amounts of isolation between subdivisions. In addition to genetic distances and F statistics, we will compute coefficients of kinship and pedigree inbreeding coefficients for the artificial populations. From previous work with another simulation model (MacCLUER et al. 1971), we expect a fair amount of variability in pedigree F. We hope to be able to determine, for certain general types of human populations, how variable these measures are likely to be under relatively constant demographic conditions, and therefore how much confidence can be placed in estimates made for actual human populations.

LITERATURE CITED

BHATTACHARYYA, A. 1946. On a measure of divergence between two multivariate populations. *Sankhya* 7:401-406.

CANNINGS, C. and A. W. F. EDWARDS. 1969. Expected genotypic frequencies in a small sample: Deviations from Hardy-Weinberg equilibrium. *Am. J. Hum. Genet.* 21: 245-247.

CAVALLI-SFORZA, L. L. and A. W. F. EDWARDS. 1967. Phylogenetic analysis. Models and estimation procedures. *Am. J. Hum. Genet.* 19:233-257.

COALE, A. J. and P. DEMENY. 1966. *Regional Model Life Tables and Stable Populations.* Princeton.

HALDANE, J. B. S. 1954. An exact test for randomness of mating. *J. Genet.* 52:631-635.

MacCLUER, J. W. 1967. Monte Carlo methods in human population genetics: A computer model incorporating age specific birth and death rates. *Am. J. Hum. Genet.*

19:303-312.

MacCLUER, J. W. and W. J. SCHULL. 1970. Frequencies of consanguineous marriage and accumulation of inbreeding in an artificial population. *Am. J. Hum. Genet.* 22: 160-175.

MacCLUER, J. W., J. V. NEEL and N. A. CHAGNON. 1971. Demographic structure of a primative population: A simulation. *Am. J. Phys. Anthro.* 35:193-208.

NEEL, J. V. and R. H. WARD. 1972. The genetic structure of a tribal population, the Yanomama Indians. VI. Analysis by F-Statistics (including a comparison with the Makiritare and Xavante). *Genetics* 72:639-666.

PURSER, A. F. 1966. Increase in heterozygote frequency with differential fertility. *Heredity* 21:322-327.

UNITED NATIONS 1965. *Population Bulletin of the United Nations No. 7-1963,* with special reference to conditions and trends of fertility in the world.

WORKMAN, P. L. 1969. The analysis of simple genetic polymorphisms. *Hum. Biol.* 41:97-114.

WORKMAN, P. L. and J. D. NISWANDER. 1970. Population studies on Southwestern Indian tribes. II. Local genetic differentiation in the Papago. *Am. J. Hum. Genet.* 22:24-49.

WRIGHT, S. 1943. Isolation by distance. *Genetics* 28:114-138.

WRIGHT, S. 1951. The genetical structure of populations. *Ann. Eugen.* 15:323-354.

APPENDIX

The measures which have been used in this analysis are arc distance, chord distance, F_{IS}, F_{IT} and F_{ST}. In the following definitions (which apply to loci with two alleles), i and j are subpopulations, n is the number of loci, and P_{ik} and q_{ik} are the frequencies of the two alleles at the kth locus in the ith subpopulation.

Arc distance:

$$ARC_{ij} = \frac{1}{n} \sum_{k=1}^{n} \frac{2}{\pi} \cos^{-1}(\sqrt{P_{ik}P_{jk}} + \sqrt{q_{ik}q_{jk}}) \qquad (1)$$

Chord distance:

$$CHORD_{ij} = \sqrt{\frac{1}{n} \sum_{k=1}^{n} \frac{8}{\pi^2}(1 - \sqrt{P_{ik}P_{jk}} - \sqrt{q_{ik}q_{jk}})} \qquad (2)$$

F_{IS}:

$$F_{IS} = \frac{1}{n} \sum_{k=1}^{n} \left(\sum_{i=1}^{m} \frac{N_i}{N} \left(1 - \frac{H_{ik}}{2p_{ik}q_{ik}} \right) \right) \quad (3)$$

where m is the number of subpopulations, N_i is the size of the ith subpopulation, N is the total population size, H_{ik} is the observed frequency of heterozygotes at locus k in the ith subpopulation.

F_{IS} (Corrected):

$$F_{IS} = \frac{1}{n} \sum_{k=1}^{n} \left(\sum_{i=1}^{m} \frac{N_i}{N} \left(1 - \frac{2N_i H_{ik}}{4N_i p_{ik}q_{ik} + H_{ik}} \right) \right) \quad (4)$$

where m, N_i, N, H_{ik} are as defined in (3). This formula incorporates the CANNINGS and EDWARDS (1969) correction for small population size.

F_{IT}:

$$F_{IT} = \frac{1}{n} \sum_{k=1}^{n} \left(1 - \frac{\overline{H}_k}{2\overline{p}_k\overline{q}_k} \right) \quad (5)$$

where $\overline{H}_k$ is the observed frequency of heterozygotes in the total population, and $\overline{p}_k$ and $\overline{q}_k$ are the allele frequencies for the entire population at the kth locus.

F_{IT} (Corrected):

$$F_{IT} = \frac{1}{n} \sum_{k=1}^{n} \left(1 - \frac{2N\overline{H}_k}{4N\overline{p}_k\overline{q}_k + \overline{H}_k} \right) \quad (6)$$

incorporating the CANNINGS and EDWARDS correction.

F_{ST}:

$$F_{ST} = \frac{1}{n} \sum_{k=1}^{n} \frac{\sigma_q^2}{\overline{p}_k\overline{q}_k} \quad (7)$$

where σ_q^2 is the variance in gene frequency between subpopulations, and $\overline{p}_k$ and $\overline{q}_k$ are as defined above. F_{ST} may also be defined in terms of the uncorrected F_{IS} and F_{IT}:

$$F_{ST} = \frac{F_{IT} - F_{IS}}{1 - F_{IS}} \quad .$$

KINSHIP BIOASSAY

N. E. Morton

Population Genetics Laboratory, University of Hawaii, Honolulu, Hawaii 96822

Heterogeneity among gene pools can be analyzed in three ways: by tests of significance, microtaxonomy, and estimation of relationship. When we consider that two gene pools must be different unless their parents were identical, it seems a sterile abuse of statistical tests to ask whether the gene pools of two groups are significantly different. However finely the anthropologist may subclassify man, the smallest category must be several orders of magnitude greater than the breeding population which concerns the geneticist, who should either be indifferent to microtaxonomic exercises, or appalled to treat our hybridizing species as a clone of bacteria. Therefore, only estimation of relationship provides an appropriate analysis of heterogeneity among gene pools.

Of the known measures of relationship, the one richest in genetic applications is MALECOT's kinship, ϕ_{ij}, defined as the probability that a pair of genes drawn at random from two gene pools i and j be identical by descent. This predicts genotype frequencies in an F_1 hybrid as a function of regional gene frequencies. No other measure of relationship, except certain functions of the ϕ_{ij}, has so simple or useful a genetic interpretation. We, therefore, take as our primary objective in studying gene pool heterogeneity the calculation of a

Population Genetics Laboratory paper No. 88. This work was supported by Grant GM 17173 from the U.S. National Institutes of Health.

symmetric matrix Φ whose $(i,j)^{th}$ element is ϕ_{ij}, knowing that any subsequent analysis, such as the measurement of isolation by distance or the estimation of genetic distance, is an operation on this matrix.

Several methods are available to predict Φ from genealogies, migration matrices, or Monte Carlo simulation. These methods are valuable, perhaps in the order given, but predictions require inductive verification. This is called *bioassay of kinship*, which subsumes all attempts to estimate kinship from observations on gene pools, independent of assumptions about genealogies, migration, or other demographic factors. So far, three kinds of data have been used: regular phenotype systems, clans or surnames, and anthropometrics.

The first attempts at phenotype bioassay considered a sample drawn from a subdivided population and simultaneously estimated gene frequencies and an average kinship for the locus. No information could be obtained from dominant-recessive pairs of genes, virtually none from ABO-like systems, and very large samples are required even with codominance. YASUDA introduced phenotype pairs, which proved much more efficient. However, the probabilities are only approximately linear in ϕ_{ij} and, as recently shown by HARPENDING, the estimates are functions both of ϕ_{ij} and α, the mean inbreeding coefficient. It therefore appears best to consider gene frequency pairs between localities. Our approach treats local gene pools as panmictic and estimates ϕ_{ij} for the hth genetic system with A_h alleles as under codominance

$$\phi_{ij} = \begin{cases} \left(\sum_{k=1}^{A_h} \hat{q}_{ki}\hat{q}_{kj}/Q_k - 1 \right) / (A_h - 1) & i \neq j \\[2em] \left(\sum_{k=1}^{A_h} E(q_{ki}^2)/Q_k - 1 \right) / (A_h - 1) & i = j \end{cases} \tag{1}$$

where

$$E(q_{ki}^2) = \frac{n_{ki}(n_{ki}-1)}{2N_i(2N_i-1)}$$

$$n_{ki} = 2N_i\hat{q}_{ki}$$

Here $\hat{q}_{ki}$ is the maximum likelihood estimate of the frequency of the kth allele in the ith population, N_i is the sample size in the ith population, and

$$Q_k = \frac{\sum\limits_i n_{ki}}{2\sum\limits_i N_i}$$

is the frequency of the kth allele in the array of populations.

The corresponding formula for surname concordance omits the factor 2 from $E(q_{ki}^2)$.

For anthropometrics (assuming that geographic variation is entirely genetic) the heritability h^2 and the intraclass correlation between populations i and j give an estimate of kinship.

A practical problem in kinship bioassay is how to combine estimates of ϕ_{ij} from different systems. Either by chance or heterogeneity in systematic pressure among systems, estimates of ϕ_{ij} must vary. We seek the average. In the absence of other knowledge, we might follow numerical taxonomy and assign equal weight to each system, regardless of number of alleles, their dominance relations, and gene frequencies. We prefer to define a weight for the hth system,

$$W_h = \frac{N_{ih}N_{jh}}{N_{ih} + N_{jh}} [1+w(k_h-1)] \qquad (2)$$

in which k_h is the amount of information about kinship per individual at $\phi = 0$ when gene frequencies are known, and $0 \le w \le 1$ is chosen so that the variance of

$$\bar{\phi}_{ij} \qquad \frac{\sum\limits_h W_h \phi_{ijh}}{\sum\limits_h W_h}$$

around the MALECOT expectation for isolation by distance is minimal.

The second practical problem in kinship bioassay is that the initial estimates of ϕ_{ij} are relative to random pairs

from the region sampled, so that values of ϕ_{ij} are negative
for a pair of populations less closely related than the
average. To refer the estimates back to ancestral gene frequencies, and so make them comparable to deductions from
genealogies, migration, or Monte Carlo simulation, we take

$$\phi'_{ij} = (\phi_{ij}-L)/(1-L) \tag{3}$$

where L is estimated as the value of ϕ_{ij} for large distances
in the region or in the limit for large distances. In our
experience, these estimates of ϕ'_{ij} have shown satisfactory
agreement with predictions of kinship when adequate data for
such predictions were available, as illustrated by FRIED-
LAENDER and HARPENDING (this volume). We take this to mean
that, over sufficiently small regions, differentiation is due
to opposing forces of genetic drift and stabilizing systematic
pressure largely from migration, with no evidence for diver-
sifying selection. This, however, may be important for larger
regions.

Two other transformations of the ϕ_{ij} have proven interesting; both are applicable to predictions as well as bioassay.
The first is the hybridity

$$\theta_{ij} = \frac{\phi_{ii} + \phi_{jj} - 2\phi_{ij}}{4 - 2\phi_{ij} - \phi_{ii} - \phi_{jj}} \doteq \frac{1}{2}\left(\frac{\phi_{ii} + \phi_{jj}}{2} - \phi_{ij}\right) \tag{4}$$

which measures the excess of heterozygositv in an F_1 relative
to an F_2 between a pair of populations; it is thus virtually
independent of regional gene frequencies. The limits of hybridity are 0 (for two populations with the same gene frequencies) and 1 (for two populations fixed for different
alleles), and so hybridity is a measure of the mean number
of allelic substitutions.

If the geographic distance between populations i and j
is d, the MALECOT expectations are

$$\phi'_{ij} = ae^{-bd} \tag{5}$$

$$\theta_{ij} = \frac{a(1-e^{-bd})}{2 - a(1+e^{-bd})} \doteq a(1-e^{-bd})/2 \tag{6}$$

Since θ_{ij} increases monotonically from zero for i = j to an asymptote at $a/2$, it is proportional to measures of genetic distance proposed by SANGVHI and others, but differs in having a simple genetic interpretation and in allowing comparison and combination of estimates.

There is, however, a different measure of genetic distance in the same units as geographic distance. Let V_i denote the ith eigenvector of a kinship matrix, where V_1 measures the genetic dispersion among populations. Let the geographic coordinates (X,Y) be regressed stepwise on the set of V_i to select the pair of most significant independent variables for each coordinate, of the form

$$X^* = A + BV_i + CV_j$$

$$Y^* = A' + B'V_m + C'V_n \tag{7}$$

Then migration is said to be isotropic if i = m and j = n, hemiisotropic if i = m but $j \neq n$, and nonisotropic if $i \neq m$ and $j \neq n$. The coordinates X^*, Y^* specify the genetic location, which may be compared with the geographic location X,Y.

The second and third eigenvectors seem in practice to provide a good estimate of X^* and Y^*, and for simplicity we propose to apply the term *genetic topology* to (7) when i = m = 2 and j = n = 3. Then the *discrepancy* between locations for the ith population is

$$D = \sqrt{(X_i-X_i^*)^2 + (Y_i-Y_i^*)^2} \tag{8}$$

and the *genetic distance* between two populations i and j is

$$G = \sqrt{(X_i^*-X_j^*)^2 + (Y_i^*-Y_j^*)^2} \tag{9}$$

both of which may be conveniently measured in km. A population that has recently migrated into a region will have a genetic location displaced toward the place of origin; an unusually inbred population will tend to be located more peripherally in the genetic space than in geographic space, and populations with high intermigration will be closer together in genetic space than geographically. We have found

genetic topology more useful and less Procrustean than
genetic trees.

The kinship matrix seems to contain all the information
about population structure. Protein evolution is an important
application of this. At the codon level a species is often
monomorphic, but unless variability is strongly reduced by
selection, the expected value of ΣQ^2 approaches zero because
of the 4^3 mutational possibilities in a codon. NEI has just
shown that under these conditions $\phi_{ij} \overset{\circ}{=} \Sigma q_i q_j$, and so the
proportion of homologous codons that are identical is a good
bioassay of kinship, which is thus equally appropriate to
local populations and to protein evolution. Kinship is,
however, not directly comparable for codons and cistrons.
If ϕ^* is the estimate for a cistron, ϕ for an average codon,
and there are N codons per cistron, then

$$\phi^* \overset{\circ}{=} \phi^N \qquad\qquad (10)$$

Since N is a large number, speciation may not involve much
change in kinship.

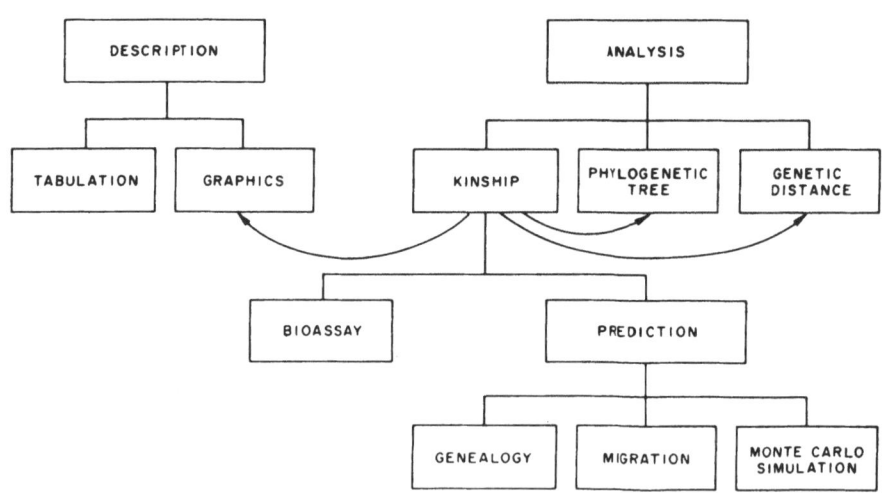

FIGURE 1.   Description and analysis of gene frequency
variation.

The central role of kinship in analysis of population structure is shown in FIGURE 1. The kinship matrix, Φ, whether bioassayed or predicted, gives a genetic topology which may be tabulated, presented graphically, or used to express biological distance in terms of hybridity or to construct phylogenetic trees. Alternative approaches are not nearly so versatile. For example, CAVALLI has suggested that a function used by him to construct phylogenetic trees,

$$F = 4[1 - \sqrt{q_i q_j} - \sqrt{(1-q_i)(1-q_j)}]$$

is an estimate of ϕ_{ij}. Actually,

$$E(q_i q_j) = q^2 - q(1-q)\theta_{ij}$$

where

$$q = (q_i + q_j)/2 \qquad .$$

Therefore

$$F = 4[1 - \sqrt{q^2 - q(1-q)\theta_{ij}} - \sqrt{(1-q)^2 - q(1-q)\theta_{ij}}] \qquad (11)$$

TABLE I

CAVALLI'S F FOR DIFFERENT VALUES OF θ AND q

			q	
θ	.01	.10	.30	.50
.0	0	0	0	0
.01	.0362	.0204	.0201	.0201
.10	--	.2936	.2099	.2053
.30	--	--	.7289	.6534
.50	--	--	--	1.1716
1.00	--	--	--	4.0000

TABLE I gives F for various values of q and θ. CAVALLI's F is a poor approximation to the hybridity, and the relation to kinship is more complicated (Equation 4).

Having completed the argument that all the information
about population structure is encoded in the kinship matrix
Φ, and in no other way (except as an enormous table of phenotype frequencies), I do not wish to obscure the practical
difficulties that remain in estimating Φ by bioassay. If
the elements of Φ are defined by (3) and (1), are these
estimates efficient and/or unbiased for a single system with
random but incomplete sampling with or without dominance?
Does (2) provide an efficient weight for combining systems?
Is (3) the appropriate transform between kinship relative to
the regional mean, and kinship relative to the expected mean?
Do (4) and (6) provide a better bioassay of the MALECOT parameters a and b than (3) and (5)? Is geographic distance in (5)
and (6) best defined as the crow flies, by the shortest road
distance, or by usual travel time? Does (9) provide a good
(i.e., heuristic) definition of genetic distance? Questions
such as these are not yet answered, and the methods of bioassay may undergo considerable improvement. Nevertheless,
it is clear that kinship is the best measure of population
structure, and kinship bioassay the only check on prediction
from genealogies, migration, or Monte Carlo simulation.

LITERATURE CITED

MORTON, N. E., S. YEE, D. E. HARRIS and R. LEW. 1971. Bio-
     assay of kinship. *J. Theor. Pop. Biol.* 2:507-524
MORTON, N. E. 1971. Reply to HARPENDING Letter to the
     Editor: Treatment of random phenotype pairs. *Amer. J.
     Hum. Genet.* 23:538-539.

A COUNTEREXAMPLE TO FITCH'S METHOD FOR MAXIMUM PARSIMONY TREES

G. William Moore

Department of Anatomy, Wayne State University College of Medicine, Detroit, Michigan 48201 U.S.A. and Pathologisches Institut, Ludwig-Aschoff-Haus, 7800 Freiburg 1. Br., Albertstrasse 19, West Germany

A major goal in numerical taxonomy over the past decade has been to discover a rapid method for finding the ancestral tree, or dendrogram, requiring the minimum number of evolutionary steps or changes, given an initial set of contemporary Operational Taxonomic Units (OTUs) for which the character states are known. Short of searching all possible dendrograms and all possible ancestral configurations for each dendrogram, the problem has never been solved in the general case. FARRIS (1970) has suggested a variety of intriguing approaches but has not proved them mathematically. ESTABROOK (1968) has solved the problem mathematically for the special case in which the CAMIN-SOKAL (1965) hypothesis is satisfied, but this special case has rather limited applications (MOORE, GOODMAN, and BARNABAS, 1973). FITCH (1971) has focused his attention on the less spectacular but more attainable goal of finding maximum parsimony ancestral character states when both the contemporary character states and the dendrogram are known. Although his method may, in many cases, find a maximum parsimony solution, it is relatively easy to demonstrate that it will not always do so.

REVIEW OF FITCH'S METHOD

As I understand the Fitch method, the amino acid sequences for the contemporary OTUs are first converted to corresponding nucleotide sequences (with allowances for ambiguity in the genetic code), and then each nucleotide

position is solved separately by a two-phase procedure: a
preliminary phase makes initial assignments of ancestral
nucleotides and a final phase "cleans up" these initial estimates. The preliminary phase of the Fitch method starts
from the contemporary OTUs and works downward in a stepwise
fashion to the root (ultimate ancestor). At each step, two
offspring join to form a single parent. The nucleotide configuration for each offspring is either input data (if the
offspring are contemporary OTUs) or constructed from a previous step. If the two offspring share nucleotides in common (nonempty intersection), then this set of common nucleotides is assigned to the parent; if the two offspring share
no nucleotides in common (empty intersection), then the set
comprising nucleotides present in either offspring (union)
is assigned to the parent. When the root has been constructed, the preliminary phase is complete. The preliminary configuration assigned to the root is considered to be final;
the final phase of the Fitch method starts from the penultimate nodes and works upward in a stepwise fashion to the contemporary OTUs. At each nonultimate node, the agreement between that node and its parent is checked. If the configurations differ (i.e., the offspring contains nucleotides not
present in the parent or vice versa), then one of three rules
(diminished ambiguity, expanded ambiguity, or encompassing
ambiguity) is used to correct the preliminary configuration
of the offspring; otherwise, the preliminary configuration
is considered final. Since no such disagreements are present in our counterexample (i.e., the preliminary and final
configurations are identical), I won't discuss these ambiguity rules in detail.

PRESENTATION OF THE COUNTEREXAMPLE

Consider the dendrogram illustrated in FIGURE 1. There
are three contemporary OTUs: OTU 1, OTU 2, and OTU 3. OTU 4
is ancestral to OTUs 1 and 2, and OTU 5 is ancestral to OTUs
3 and 4. Suppose OTU 1 is known to have the amino acid phenyl-
alanine (PHE) in some alignment position, and OTUs 2 and 3 are
known to have amino acid leucine (LEU) in the same alignment
position. The first step in Fitch's method is to find which
codons (nucleotide triplets) correspond to each of the known
amino acids. In this case, PHE has codons UUC and UUU whereas LEU has codons CUA, CUC, CUG, CUU, UUA, and UUG (FIGURE 2).
The next step in Fitch's method is to separate the trees in
FIGURE 2 into three parallel trees corresponding to positions
I, II, and III on the codon. The result of this separation

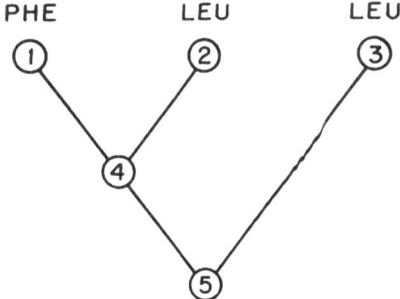

FIGURE 1. OTU numbers are circled. The amino acids for contemporary OTUs (1, 2, and 3) are known and indicated by appropriate three-letter codes.

(PHE)	(LEU)	(LEU)
	CUA	CUA
	CUC	CUC
	CUG	CUG
	CUU	CUU
UUC	UUA	UUA
UUU	UUG	UUG

FIGURE 2. Nucleotide codons corresponding to the known amino acids for the dendrogram of FIGURE 1.

is shown in FIGURE 3. In position I, OTU 1 has only nucleotide U, whereas OTUs 2 and 3 have nucleotides C and U. In position II, all three OTUs have only nucleotide U. In position III, OTU 1 has nucleotides C and U, whereas OTUs 2 and 3 have all four nucleotides, A, C, G, and U.

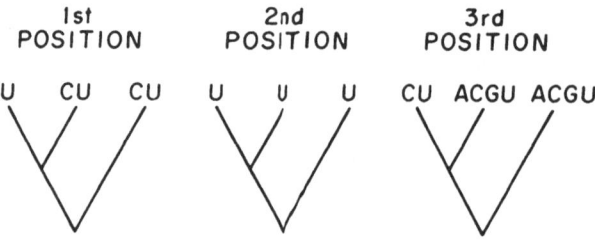

FIGURE 3.   Separation of nucleotides for the codon dendrograms of FIGURE 2.

All three positions may be solved completely in the preliminary phase by use of the intersection rule. This solution procedure gives the following result (FIGURE 4).

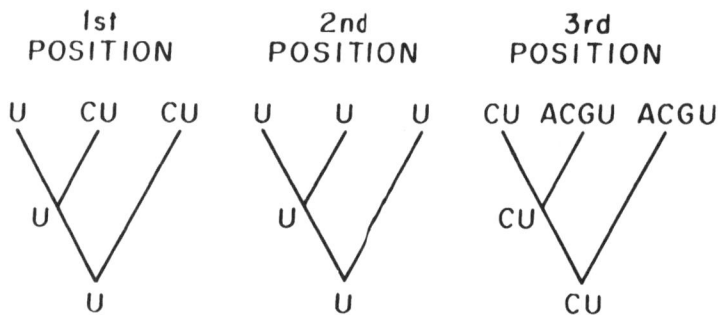

FIGURE 4.   Solution of the separate nucleotide positions using Fitch's method for the nucleotide dendrograms of FIGURE 3.

In positions I and II, OTUs 4 and 5 have only nucleotide U. In position III, OTUs 4 and 5 have nucleotides C and U. Since the penultimate node always agrees with the root, no final phase preprocessing is required. When the parallel trees at positions I, II, and III have been reassembled, OTUs 4 and 5 have UUC and UUU as possible codons (FIGURE 5).

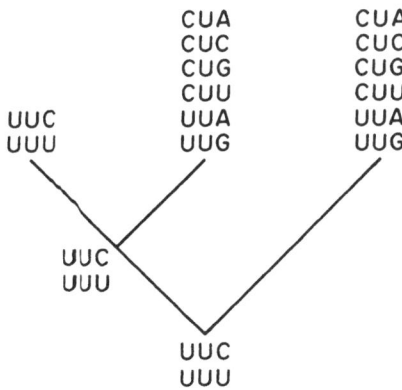

FIGURE 5. The separate nucleotide positions of FIGURE 4 have been reassembled to provide Fitch codon solutions.

Each pair of neighboring OTUs in a dendrogram is connected by a <u>link</u>. To each link in a dendrogram, there is a non-negative integer called its <u>linklength</u>. The linklength of a link is the number of nonmatching nucleotide positions for the two OTUs at either end of the link. The <u>length</u> of an entire dendrogram is the sum of linklengths over all links in the dendrogram. A <u>maximum parsimony solution</u> of a dendrogram is a choice of codons for all OTUs on the dendrogram such that the length is minimal. There are four possible ways to permute the codons permitted by FIGURE 5 to give a tree of length two (FIGURE 6). There is no way to permute the codons of FIGURE 5 to give a tree of length less than two. There are six trees of length one (not included among the Fitch possibilities) whose contemporary codons are consistent with the known amino acids for OTUs 1, 2, and 3 (FIGURE 7). In other words, the Fitch method has eliminated all the maximum parsimony solutions and left behind only nonparsimony solutions.

DISCUSSION

Fitch's method does not always eliminate the maximum parsimony solutions, but the fact that such a simple example

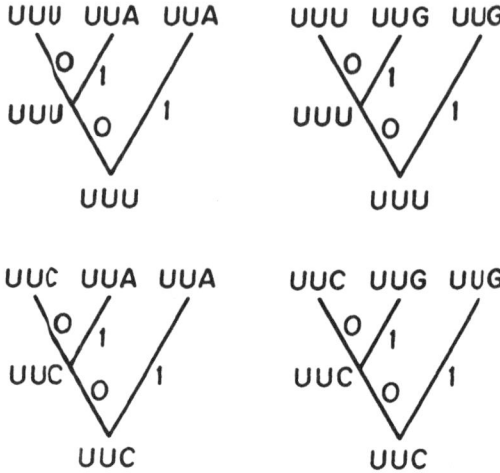

FIGURE 6. There are four ways to permute the codons permitted by the Fitch method (FIGURE 5) to give a tree of length two, as displayed above. There is no way to permute these codons to give a tree of length less than two. Individual link-lengths are displayed to the right of each link.

eludes the method should make one cautious about drawing serious conclusions from results so derived. The fact that Fitch's method missed the true solution for the above example by only a single mutation is not comforting, because it is easy to construct more complex counterexamples for which Fitch's method misses the true solution by a substantial margin. One can always hope that "real data" are benign enough such that Fitch's method comes relatively close to the maximum parsimony solution, but one can never be sure.

A more serious shortcoming in Fitch's method is its apparent tendency to underestimate the true number of mutations in a so-called maximum parsimony solution. According to Fitch's rules for reconstructing mutation lengths, any tree which has been solved entirely by the intersection rule in the preliminary phase has a total length of zero. Yet for the example herein developed, any tree with the

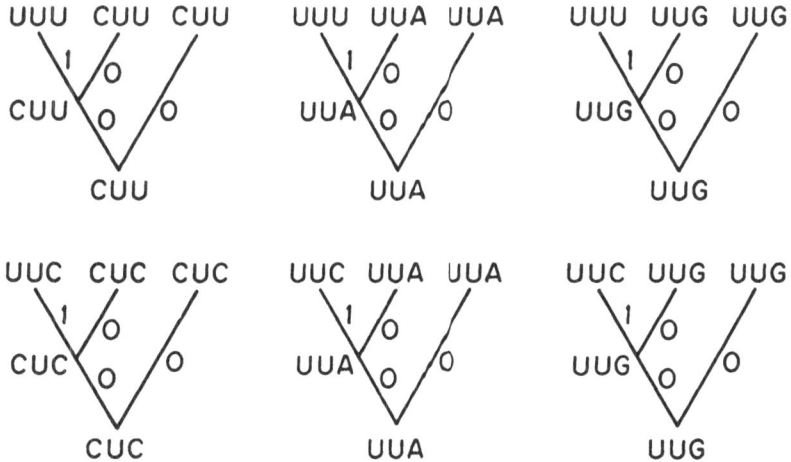

FIGURE 7. There are six trees on length one, not included
among the Fitch possibilities, whose contemporary codons
are consistent with the known amino acids given in FIGURE 1.
Individual linklengths are displayed to the right of each
link.

nucleotides specified by Fitch's method must have a length
of at least two, and even the true maximum parsimony solutions have length one. As before, the fact that Fitch's
method gives a "near miss" to the correct answer is not
consoling, since much worse counterexamples can easily be
constructed. Since Fitch's method cannot be counted upon
to estimate the correct mutation length, it is of limited
interest in distinguishing a "correct dendrogram topology"
(which permits the least mutation length of all possible
dendrogram topologies) from alternatives.

My colleagues and I have proved three maximum parsimony
theorems from which we have developed a computer program
capable of solving the ancestral amino acid sequence problem for a given dendrogram topology (MOORE, BARNABAS, and
GOODMAN, 1973). By using mathematically proven theorems
as the basis for our method we have designed a method safe
from counterexamples.

LITERATURE CITED

CAMIN, J. H. and R. R. SOKAL. 1965. A method for deducing branching sequences in phylogeny. *Evolution* 19:311-326.

ESTABROOK, G. F. 1968. A general solution in partial orders for the Camin-Sokal model in phylogeny. *J. Theor. Biol.* 21:421-438.

FARRIS, J. S. 1970. Methods for computing Wagner trees. *Syst. Zool.* 19:83-92.

FITCH, W. M. 1971. Toward defining the course of evolution: minimum change for a specific tree topology. *Syst. Zool.* 20:406-416.

MOORE, G. W., J. BARNABAS and M. GOODMAN. 1973. A method for constructing maximum parsimony ancestral amino acid sequences on a given network. *J. Theor. Biol.* 38:459-485.

MOORE, G. W., M. GOODMAN and J. BARNABAS. 1973. An iterative approach from the standpoint of the additive hypothesis to the dendrogram problem posed by molecular data sets. *J. Theor. Biol.* 38:423-457.

ADDENDUM: A COUNTEREXAMPLE TO FITCH'S METHOD FOR MAXIMUM PARSIMONY TREES

Subsequent to my receipt of his preliminary manuscript, Dr. Fitch informed me of a modification of the manuscript which will appear in the published version in *Systematic Zoology*. Since I was unaware of this modification at the time of the Paris congress, I should like to comment on it now. In Dr. Fitch's words:

> One additional caveat is in order when translating amino acid sequences into codon sequences, namely, a selection must be made between the codons A.C. (CU) and U.C. (ACGU) for serine, A.G. (AG) and C.G. (ACGU) for arginine, and U.U. (AG) and C.U. (ACGU) for leucine. Any attempt at total ambiguity leads to such cases as that A.C.A. (threonine), U.G.U. (cysteine) or others are present when in fact only serine is present. This in turn could lead to other errors. A computer procedure is available for translating amino acids into codons that selects the codons for serine, arginine, and leucine that are most likely to give the fewest mutations.

Limitation of the codons permitted for a particular amino acid does indeed vitiate the counterexample presented above, but it does not free Fitch's method from all counterexamples. Consider the more complex problem presented in FIGURE 8. The amino acid ARG (alluded to in Fitch's revision) is found twice among the contemporary amino acids. There are two maximum parsimony solutions corresponding to this initial collection of amino acids (FIGURE 9), neither of which permits the same codon to be used for ARG. That is, the codon for the left ARG codon must always come from the C.G. (ACGU) group, whereas the right ARG codon must always come from the A.G. (AG) group. In this particular example, there may be some way to assign one group of ARG codons to one region of the tree and the other group of ARG codons to the rest of the tree, but the specifics of such a piecewise codon assignment procedure are certainly not clear in Dr. Fitch's revised manuscript.

113

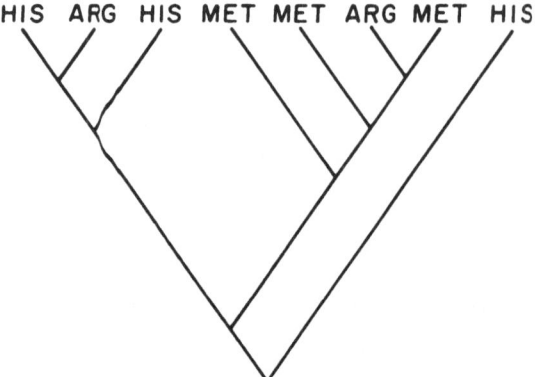

FIGURE 8.   Another counterexample.

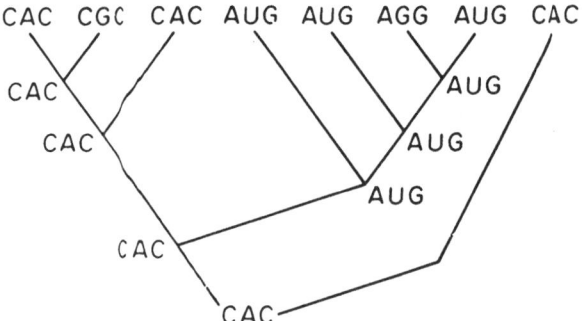

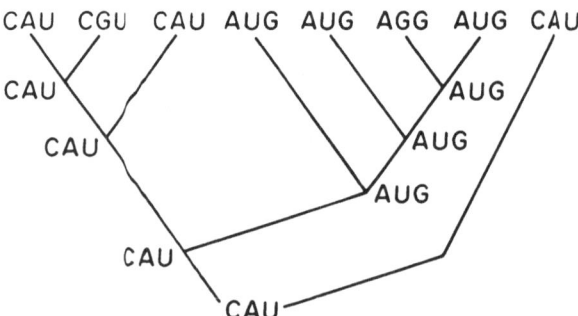

FIGURE 9.   Two maximum parsimony solutions for the tree in
FIGURE 8.   Neither permits the same codon for ARG.

The value of Dr. Fitch's revision is also unclear in examples such as that of FIGURE 10, where the sixteen maximum parsimony solutions (FIGURE 11) include not only trees for which the choice of SER codon-groups (either the A.G. (CU) group or the U.C. (ACGU) group) varies within the same tree, but include as well pairs of solutions for which the SER codon-group at a particular OTU for one solution differs from the SER codon-group in the other solution at the same OTU. I find it difficult to imagine a "most likely"

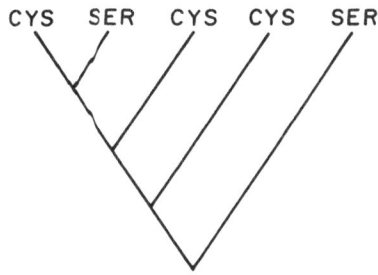

FIGURE 10. A tree with two SER's.

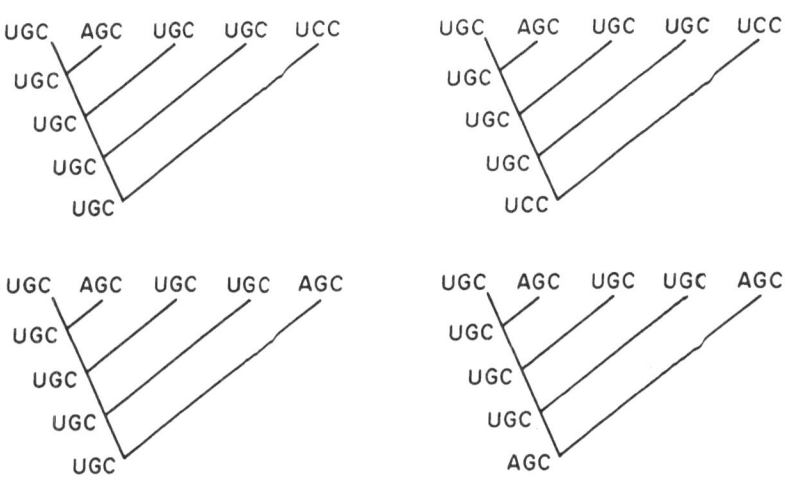

FIGURE 11. Eight of the 16 minimum parsimony solutions.
(FIGURE 11 continued on following page.)

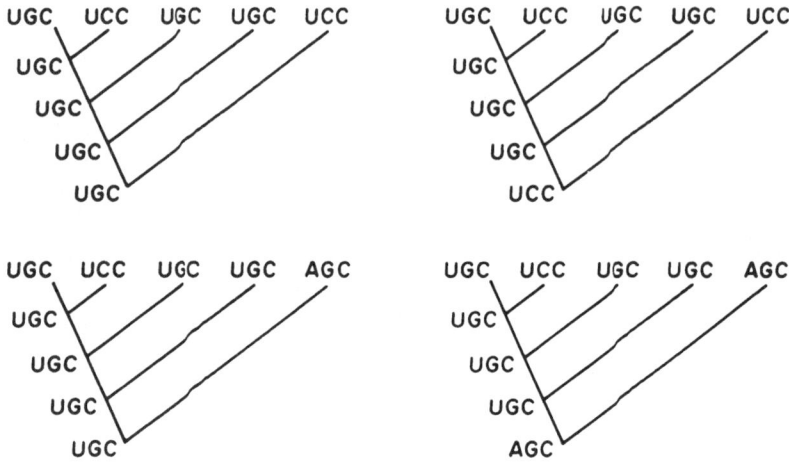

FIGURE 11.   Eight of the 16 minimum parsimony solutions.
              (Continued from previous page.)

way of assigning a single SER codon-group to a particular
OTU, when in fact all possible codon-group assignments may
correspond to an acceptable solution.

RESPONSE TO THE PAPER OF DR. MOORE

Walter M. Fitch

Department of Physiological Chemistry
University of Wisconsin
Madison, Wisconsin 53706

I should begin by stating that I am very sorry that I
could not attend the workshop in which Dr. Morton kindly in-
vited me to participate. As a consequence of my absence I
must indicate my appreciation to Drs. Morton and Crow, as
organizer and moderator-editor, for asking me to respond to
Dr. Moore's remarks, and especially to express my sincerest
thanks to Dr. Moore in sending me a copy of his paper and,
subsequently, a copy of his addendum.

I shall address myself only to Dr. Moore's addendum
since his earlier remarks were based upon an assumption that
in applying my method to real data I utilized a degree of
codon ambiguity that was not in fact the case. However,
Dr. Moore's error was all my fault since the manuscript I
originally sent him did not state the crucial point that in
practice I translated amino acids into codons so that ambiguity occurred only in the third nucleotide position. My
failure to include this point was the result of my having no
real intention of dealing with that translation problem. As
the last sentence of my introduction states, "Thus, <u>given a
set of descendent nucleotide sequences</u> and a topology pre-
sumed to describe their ancestral relationships, one can
set forth: (a) the exact number of nucleotide replacements
that are the minimum necessary to account for the descent of
those sequences from a common ancestor, (b) all possible ancestral sequences at each node that are consistent with that
minimum; [plus two more points; underscoring added]". Thus
my method starts with the assumption that we have a nucleotide

117

sequence.

Dr. Moore's addendum shows, in FIGURES 9 and 11, eigh-
teen examples, each of which contains a specified tree and
a specific set of nucleotide sequences for each descendent.
My method would do for each of those trees precisely what
Dr. Moore has done and so we are in complete agreement on all
those points.

Dr. Moore also points out (quite correctly) that if one
begins with amino acids, one cannot easily be sure which codons should be assigned and, more specifically, that for a
most parsimonious solution, different codons may be absolutely
required for the same amino acid appearing in distantly related taxa. That is fine, but it involves a question I did
not presume to attack, *viz*, what are the nucleotide sequences
in the genes, given only the amino acid sequences in the gene
products? A legitimate counterexample must meet all the underlying assumptions but possess a solution that the proposed algorithm will not find. The present so-called counterexamples
do not meet the requirement: "given a set of descendent nucleotide sequences". Nevertheless, Dr. Moore has raised a most important question, the answer to which is necessary for the op-
timal utilization of amino acid sequences for evolutionary
studies and I am glad that he has raised it. More than that,
I am pleased that his efforts will have made clearer to every-
one what my procedure is and is not intended to do.

There is, however, one instance where the most parsimonious solution for each of three nucleotide positions may
combine to give a biologically unreasonable solution. Any-
time three nodes of the tree are connected to each other
through a single fourth node and those three nodes have the
amino acids tyrosine, tryptophan (or a leucine whose codon
is UUR), and one of three amino acids, glutamate, glutamine
or lysine, the most parsimonious solution (three mutations)
requires the fourth (intermediate) node to possess the codon
UAG which is a chain terminating codon and therefore biologically very improbable as an ancestral state. The accompanying
FIGURE shows one such example. There is one mutation on
each leg, the nucleotide changed as a result of that mutation
being shown by underlining. Such a case occurs in position
91 of beta hemoglobin where the presently known sequences
have lysine (AAR) in that position in the two lampreys,
tyrosine (UAY) in the frog and leucine (UUR) in all others.
Since the terminating UAR is part of the most parsimonious

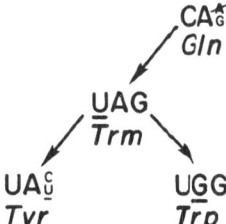

FIGURE: An example where the most parsimonious solution is
a terminating codon.

solution, an additional mutation is to be anticipated. In
that case leucine could just as well be coded for by CUX.

ERROR IN THE RECONSTRUCTION OF EVOLUTIONARY TREES

Kenneth K. Kidd, Paola Astolfi and
L. L. Cavalli-Sforza

Department of Genetics, Stanford University
School of Medicine, Stanford, California 94305
(K.K. and L.L.C.-S.), and Istituto di Genetica,
Universita di Pavia, Pavia, 27100, Italy

Reconstruction of the evolutionary history of organisms in the form of phylogenetic trees has been popular since Darwin's time. In the last decades, some work has been devoted to trying to put these methods on a quantitative basis. Sometimes these methods are applied to the reconstruction of the differentiation between species; only fission processes are involved here, in agreement with the definition of a species. At other times, these methods have been concerned with the reconstruction of the differentiation within species; migration and exchange of genes is at least potentially possible here, and a complete description should attempt to consider episodes of fusion as well as fission. The methods with which we have been concerned are applicable to gene frequency data (CAVALLI-SFORZA and EDWARDS 1967, KIDD and SGARAMELLA-ZONTA 1971). These methods consider within-species differentiation and so far are applicable only to fission processes. This has always been recognized as a limitation. On the other hand, a judicious choice of populations that are not very closely related, so that migration between them

This work was supported by a National Institutes of Health Postdoctoral Fellowship to K.K.K. and by the Stanford-Pavia Exchange Program under the National Science Foundation Grant GB-7785. The use of computer facilities at the Universita di Pavia was also supported by the Laboratorio di Genetica Biochimia ed Evoluzionistica di Pavia del Consiglio Nazionale delle Ricerche.

121

is relatively small, was thought to be a sufficient guarantee
that the methods could still be applied in spite of the fact
that some migration and fusion processes might have been going on. This was, for instance, the case of the first application to 15 human groups selected to represent the human species
(CAVALLI-SFORZA and EDWARDS 1964). Considerations in the choice
of the populations selected were then more of a geographical
nature. In other cases, such as in cattle, enough is known
of the history of some breeds that the assumption of a pure
fission process can be largely satisfied, making the results
more representative of the actual breed histories (KIDD and
SGARAMELLA-ZONTA 1972, KIDD and PIRCHNER 1971).

The reconstruction of phylogeny is an ambitious task,
and should certainly take account of all available elements:
historical, geographical, biological, cultural, etc. The
methods we have suggested use gene frequency data, which we
believe provide the strongest type of phylogenetic evidence.
It is, in any case, obvious that agreement with all other
sources of data should eventually be reached and possible
discrepancies explained. We will not insist, in this paper,
on the validity of the biological assumptions on which our
methods are based, except for noting that a minor formal
point is easily resolved. The methods we have been using
reconstruct only bifurcation, and there certainly were times
in evolutionary history where more complex subdivisions than
simple bifurcations have taken place. We should, perhaps,
reiterate here the almost trivial consideration that two
closely following bifurcations are practically indistinguishable from a trifurcation. A point of more importance is
that the choice of the scale used for measuring genetic distances between the populations examined is a vital one. There
has been an explosion of genetic distance measurements recently, and we only want to stress here the fact that those
measurements which we believe are valid are those which come
closer to the mathematical model which we employ in the analysis. A few more specific comments will be found in what
follows.

It is interesting that the most recent and thorough
study of the origin of human races (KIDD 1973) confirmed
the early phylogenetic tree suggested by CAVALLI-SFORZA and
EDWARDS (1964), expressing close general agreement with the
relationships shown by that tree, although the source of the
information is, at least in part, independent since entirely
different populations and some different genetic loci were

used. The history of the early separation of human races
is, however, vague, and even agreement with the conclusions
of well known anthropologists (e.g., COON 1965) could not
bring much weight to the validity of the methods themselves.
Of more importance in this respect is that WARD and NEEL
(1970) have shown that tree analysis of a group of Makiritare
village populations, whose recent history of fission and
fusion was known, gave rather faithful reconstruction of
their history. This suggests that the methods give satisfactory results even when some of the assumptions underlying
the applications of the methods are violated. Thus it is
possible that the methods are more robust than we would have
anticipated at first.

Still leaving aside the validity of the biological
assumptions underlying the method, the fact remains that
the statistical and mathematical problems raised by the reconstruction of phylogenetic trees have so far been solved
with methods known to be approximate, in spite of the fact
that they demand a considerable amount of computer work.
EDWARDS (1970) has shown that the maximum likelihood solution for what appears to be the simplest model (Brownian
motion/Yule process) is intractable even by computer analysis. KIDD and SGARAMELLA-ZONTA (1971) have discussed
some of the sources of errors in the least squares and
minimum path methods that had been suggested earlier. In
general, the magnitude of these errors cannot be directly
estimated, and hence the statistical reliability of the
results obtained cannot yet be ascertained.

As a theoretical analysis seems difficult, recourse
was made to simulation. KIDD and CAVALLI-SFORZA (1971)
reported the results of a simulation study designed to
quantify the errors involved in estimating phylogenetic
trees and to study the relative efficacy of some different methods. In that study, characters underwent a random walk with three fissions resulting in four final
populations; the various methods were then used on the
final character values to attempt to estimate the correct
relationships of those four populations.

The methods tried varied significantly in efficacy.
The one using the quantity Σe^2 (minimized in a least
squares solution) was consistently inferior to the other
methods. It was shown earlier (KIDD and SGARAMELLA-ZONTA
1971) that this method is very closely associated with a

similar one employed by FITCH and MARGOLIASH (1967). Of all
other methods tested, none was consistently superior. In particular, the methods used were based on correlation coefficients (KIDD and CAVALLI-SFORZA 1971), cluster analysis
(EDWARDS and CAVALLI-SFORZA 1965), minimum path (EDWARDS 1969),
and least squares using the statistic LS length (KIDD and
SGARAMELLA-ZONTA 1971). It is worth noting that this last
method gives results practically indistinguishable from those
obtained by choosing the tree with the smallest value of the
quantity Σe^2, but adding the restriction that trees contain-
ing negative segments should be discarded. This double criterion was the method used in the early work of EDWARDS and
CAVALLI-SFORZA. An example of that simulation is given in
FIGURE 1.

We are now extending simulation studies to trees of 6
and 15 populations. Six populations is the maximum for which
all possible unrooted trees (105) can be quickly and econom-
ically studied. Fifteen is the maximum which can be econom-
ically studied by the published method of cluster analysis.
(It is worth adding that unpublished recent work has extended
the maximum number for cluster analysis to 40.) With fifteen
populations, however, the number of different trees is so
large that an exhaustive analysis by the other methods is
currently impossible. We are interested in comparing the
methods under these more trying conditions and, for those
that also estimate segment lengths, ascertaining the accuracy
as well as the possible biases of their estimation. If it
can be assumed that evolutionary rates are constant, segment
lengths measured as genetic distance should supply reliable
estimates of the corresponding time intervals: this is obviously a point of importance in the quantitative study of
evolution. The results presented here are preliminary in
that most are based on only 20 simulated trees; we are currently expanding the study to a total of 50 simulated trees
for each analysis.

SIMULATION METHOD

We have generated trees according to a Yule process.
The time intervals between splits, following the initial
split at time zero, are first selected using

$$T_n = \frac{-\log R}{n}, \qquad 2 \leq n \leq N$$

where

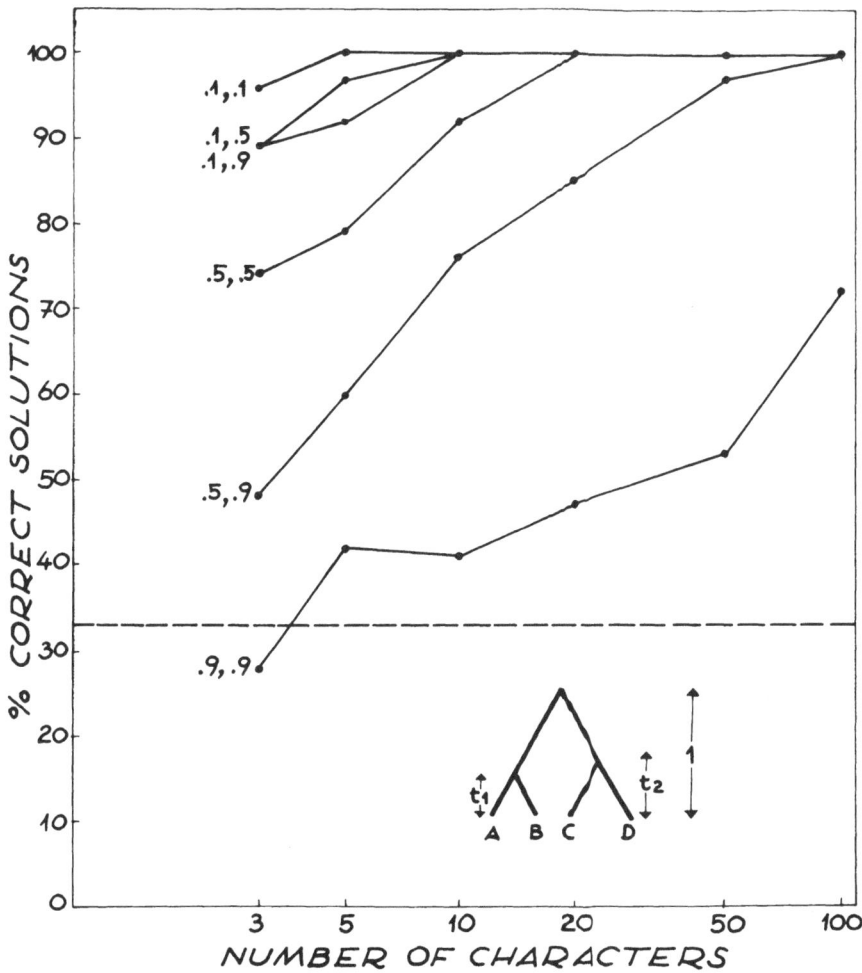

FIGURE 1. Probability of correct tree reconstruction for 4
populations using LS length. Each curve corresponds to the
topology inset using the branching times, t_1 and t_2, given
at the left. Each point represents the results of at least
100 independently generated trees. Random chance alone gives
a probability of one-third, indicated by the dashed line.
Correct reconstruction is clearly a function of both number
of characters and the relative degree of separation of the
populations. (From data in KIDD and CAVALLI-SFORZA, 1971.)

R   =   random number between zero and one with uniform
          distribution

T_n =   length of the interval during which there are n
          populations

N   =   final number of populations

The tree is stopped at the time the $(N+1)^{th}$ population would
be formed. The topology is generated by randomly selecting,
at the end of each interval, one of the n populations to
split into two.

The characters are generated by the same method previously
used (KIDD and CAVALLI-SFORZA 1971). At each splitting time
all characters are "updated" by adding to the previous character value a random normal variate with zero mean and standard
deviation equal to the square root of the time interval since
the last split. All characters are initialized to zero at the
beginning of the tree; two sibling populations are given the
same character values at the time of their split but then
"drift" (i.e. undergo Brownian motion) independently, with
the updating procedure already described. The random numbers
actually used were the pseudorandom numbers generated by the
programs using the IBM subroutines RANDU for the random numbers and GAUSS for the normal variates.

Thus, a population may be considered as a point in a
multidimensional space with each character equated to one
orthogonal axis and the character values defining the position of the point. Distances between populations are calculated as the straight line distances between these points
in a Euclidean space. These distances thus approximate the
E distances (EDWARDS 1971) calculated on gene frequencies.

The final output for each tree consists of the tree form
with final populations labeled, the real segment lengths (in
"time" units) for all segments, the character values for the
final populations, and the Euclidean distances between the
populations.

THE ANALYSIS

Unless otherwise specified the computer programs and
statistics used are as described in KIDD and SGARAMELLA-ZONTA

(1971).

Methods for Selection of Tree Form

Cluster Analysis (CA). We used the method of EDWARDS
and CAVALLI-SFORZA (1965) and examined all $2^{n-1} - 1$ possible
partitions into two subsets at each stage of the analysis;
one tree results from taking the best partition at each
stage.

Least Squares (LS). We used two least squares programs:
one examines all possible trees (used for trees of 6 populations), and the other modifies initial input trees searching
for a better fit (used for trees of 15 populations). In
both cases, the statistic LS length is used to compare trees.
For 6-population trees, two different distances were used.
The results are presented separately for least squares using
the Euclidean distances, LS(E), and for least squares using
the square of those distances, LS(sq).

Minimum Path (MP). We used the minimum path program to
evaluate all possible trees for the 6-population trees. The
best tree was taken as the one with smallest MP length.

Estimation of Segment Lengths

This question is to some extent independent from the
problem of reconstruction of the correct topology. We compared the real segment lengths generated by the simulation
of a Yule process with the estimated segment lengths obtained
when the correct topology is solved using the various methods,
LS(E), LS(sq), and MP.

In addition to LS and MP on the Euclidean distances, LS
estimates were obtained using the mean distance (averaged
over the characters) and the mean squared distance (identical
to the squared distance divided by 20, the number of characters).

RESULTS

Six-Population Trees

It is immediately clear from the first column of results

TABLE   I

RESULTS FOR TREES OF 6 POPULATIONS

METHOD	NUMBER OF TREES EXAMINED	PER CENT CORRECT SOLUTIONS	NUMBER OF TOPO-LOGICAL CHANGES FROM BEST TREE TO CORRECT ONE		RANK OF CORRECT TREE	
			MEAN ±	STANDARD ERROR	MEAN ±	STANDARD ERROR
LS(E)	20	45	0.75	.18	4.45	1.22
LS(sq)	20	45	0.85	.20	9.85	3.34
MP	20	45	1.05	.27	5.45	1.45
CA	40	50 (unrooted)	.85	.18	--	--
		35 (rooted)				

For the first three methods all possible trees were evaluated.
The statistical rank of the correct tree, and the topological
similarity of the correct tree to the statistically best tree,
were used to compare the methods. Cluster analysis produces
only one tree, so could not be compared by rank; however, it
does produce rooted solutions. Cluster analysis appears
slightly superior to LS(E); the other two methods are inferior.

in TABLE I that with 20 characters we get the correct solution
only about half the time no matter which method is used; we
cannot discriminate among the methods on this basis. Topological differences between the best tree (by each method) and
the true tree can be measured as the number of changes needed
to transform one tree into another. A change is the transi-
tion from a given topology to one of the other two possible
arrangements around a specific segment (KIDD and SGARAMELLA-
ZONTA 1971). The mean and its standard error for this
"statistic" are given in TABLE I. While the means show differences suggesting that LS(E) is best and MP is worst, the
standard errors are sufficiently large that we cannot consider
the difference in this "statistic" to be significant. A
statistical difference between the best tree and the true tree
can be measured as the rank of the correct tree by either the
statistic LS length or the statistic MP length. One must use

rank since the absolute values of each statistic depend on
the data and method used. The mean rank and its standard
error are also given in TABLE I. Again the means favor LS(E),
but here the differences may be significant. Pairwise differences for the three methods show no significant differences
when the t test is used. However, the distributions are not
normal. The sign test shows LS(E) significantly better than
LS(sq) with p about equal to .001. The ranked sign test for
the other two comparisons shows no significance if allowance
is made for multiple tests. Thus, we are as yet unable to
show significant differences among the methods, although we
have a strong suggestion that LS(E) is best.

Fifteen-Population Trees

There are approximately 10^{13} different ways of relating
fifteen populations with a bifurcating tree. We used CA to
produce a tree from the data and examined a few likely trees
by LS(E) using the change procedure described by KIDD and
SGARAMELLA-ZONTA (1971). The CA tree was never entirely
correct, but the first partition into two groups corresponded
to the initial split (root) in 45% of the trees examined.
While this may seem low, it is much better than chance alone,
since there are $2^{14} - 1$ possible splits. As a measure of
topological similarity, we determined the number of changes
between the trees as before. The CA tree was, on average,
4.60 changes from the true tree. The best tree, of the few
examined by LS(E), was also never the correct one -- it always
had a lower statistical value than either the true tree or the
CA tree. The number of changes between the true and "best"
(by LS length) was, on average, 4.05. With the number of
changes as the criterion LS(E) was better than CA, but again
the difference was not significant.

Since only a fraction of all possible trees was examined
by least squares, we cannot be sure that the statistically
best tree was evaluated and cannot compare ranks. We have
therefore based our statistical comparisons on deviations
from the mean. Since KIDD and SGARAMELLA-ZONTA (1971) showed
that the statistics LS length and MP length might be approximated by a normal distribution, we took for each of the 20
simulated data sets a random sample of trees, evaluated them,
and calculated a mean and standard deviation for the statistic
LS length. The standard normal deviate values were then calculated for the LS length of the tree with the smallest value

(the "best" found by LS(E)), the CA tree, and the true tree.
Mean values over the 20 replicates were -7.813 for the "best"
trees, -7.410 for the CA trees, and -7.035 for the correct
trees. The immediately evident aspect of these values is
that they are all more than 7 standard deviations below the
mean; while LS length does not give the lowest value to the
correct tree under these conditions, taking the lowest value
found gives a crude approximation. Because of the errors in
estimating each standard error, plus those in taking the
means, a significance test is difficult. These three means
are not likely to be significantly different at this point
in our study. By the sign test, however, this order is
highly significant. An interpretation is difficult, since
both methods were "better" than the correct tree, but the
LS(E) method, which was further statistically from the true
tree, was closer topologically.

Segment Length Estimation

In the Yule/Poisson process the variance expected between
two populations drifting independently is equal to $\sigma^2 t$ where
t is total time of separation. In our simulation the variance of the normal variates used to simulate each character
had $\sigma^2 = 1$, so that the variance expected between two populations is expected to be $t = 2t'$, where t' refers to the
time since separation and the factor of 2 is due to the fact
that the evolutionary process goes on independently in the
two branches leading to the two populations after the split.

On the other hand, the square of the distance between
the two populations for one character is but twice the variance. We thus expect the square of the distance between two
populations for one character to be simply equal to the total
time separation since the last split; that is, $2t'$. When the
squared distance is computed for 20 independent characters
and the values are averaged, the expected mean squared distance remains the same as before, namely, equal to the value
t.

We have, therefore, taken the segment lengths estimated
by the various methods using not only the mean of the squared
distances, but also the other measurements of distance which
have been suggested and used in this paper. The results are
given in TABLE II. The study of the linear regression of
estimated segment lengths in the true topologies shows that

TABLE II

RESULTS OF ESTIMATION OF SEGMENT LENGTHS

METHOD AND DISTANCE MEASURE*	6-POPULATION TREES		15-POPULATION TREES	
	CORRELATION COEFFICIENT	REGRESSION	CORRELATION COEFFICIENT	REGRESSION
$\dfrac{LS(E)}{\sqrt{\Sigma d^2}}$	.79	$S=.884+1.583 \cdot T$	.69	$S=.747+1.467 \cdot T$
$\dfrac{LS(\text{mean})}{\Sigma d/20}$	.78	$S=.165+.276 \cdot T$	.68	$S=.135+.267 \cdot T$
$\dfrac{LS(\text{mean squared distance})}{\Sigma d^2/20}$	.81	$S=.001+1.024 \cdot T$	.78	$S=.042+.895 \cdot T$
$\dfrac{MP}{\sqrt{\Sigma d^2}}$	.80	$S=1.286+1.734 \cdot T$	.77	$S=1.137+1.783 \cdot T$

*The distance is calculated for a pair of populations, i
and j, with summation over all k characters (k = 20)
and with $d_{ijk} = |x_{ik} - x_{jk}|$, where x_{ik} is the value
of the ith population for the kth character.

S equals estimated length of segment, and T equals true length
of segment.

only when we use mean squared distances for computations by
least squares, as indicated in the first line, do we come
close to the expected proportionality between S and T, with
an expected proportionality constant of 1. That is, S = T.
All other methods used gave correlations that were clearly
curvilinear (convex upward) and somewhat smaller. These results, therefore, indicate that only if we choose the proper
measurement of distance can we hope to estimate segment
lengths that are proportional to actual time. All other

methods produce biases in the evaluation of time lengths.
With all methods except the one expected to be correct, given
in the first line, long segments seen to be underestimated,
on average. Since this work will be enlarged and more trees
are now being examined, we will further analyze this point
in the near future. It may be mentioned that here, as well
as in other similar situations, there are difficulties in
applying exact tests of significance because of the non-
independence of segments obtained in the same tree.

DISCUSSION

The probability of finding the correct unrooted tree by
chance, when there are only 6 populations, is just slightly
less than 1%. Thus, all of our methods have given the correct tree much more often than by chance alone, and, in fact,
all have given the correct topology about half the time.
These results were obtained with 20 characters, and we cannot
yet say how many characters would be necessary to increase
the probability of reaching the correct tree to a value closer
to 100%. It should be noted, however, that the error of reconstruction is on average a little less than one change,
which means that the correct tree differs from the estimated
one only by the fact that two neighboring populations are
somehow interchanged. This is, perhaps, not too bad an approximation. Though it is difficult to judge their significance, there are differences among the methods. The correct
tree is, on average, closer in rank to the statistically best
tree by LS(E) than by LS(sq) or by MP. The statistically best
tree has, on average, greater topological similarity to the
correct tree when obtained by LS(E) than when obtained by the
other methods, but the differences are small and the significance relatively doubtful.

With trees of 15 populations, the probability of obtaining the correct unrooted tree by chance alone is about 10^{-13}.
It is impossible to examine all the 7.9×10^{12} different trees
to be certain of finding the correct tree. Indeed, in 20
trials the correct tree has never been obtained from CA, nor
has it been statistically best by the other three methods.
However, the criterion chosen as goodness of fit, LS length,
was seven standard deviations below the mean of the same value
computed for random trees and very close to the value for the
true tree. Also, the "best" tree by LS(E) and the CA tree
are both topologically very similar to the true tree, though

the LS(E) tree seems most similar. As an indication of the
degree of improvement over chance that a difference of 4-5
changes represents, we calculated the average number of changes
required to convert one randomly generated tree into another.
On 10 pairs of these random trees we found that an average of
24.8 changes was required to convert one tree into the other.
However, since there is no unique way of performing these
changes, we are not certain that the absolute minimum number
was found in each case. We are certain, however, that the
mean could not be much lower than the value we found, since
several independent conversions were made for each pair and
the lowest value taken to calculate the mean.

The segment lengths seem to be most accurately estimated
using the mean squared distance. This is theoretically expected from our character generation procedure, but is in
some contrast to the estimation of the correct topology. In
that case, LS(E) was always as good as or better than LS(sq).
Thus, it is possible that the best method for estimating segment lengths is not the same as that for inferring the right
topology, but this difficulty may be overcome by repeating
the computation of segment length with LS(sq) once the best
tree has been obtained by CA or LS(E). Clarification must
await additional data.

CONCLUSIONS

The use of tree analyses has been criticized by MORTON
(1974). However, we feel that in many cases population histories can be approximated by a tree structure and that such
analyses are then appropriate. The present results show that
in the ideal case of a Brownian motion/Yule process our methods
do give a highly significant improvement over chance in reconstructing the tree. The accuracy would be improved if more
characters were used, but 20 independent characters is approximately the number that have been used in studies of real populations. With 6 populations they seem to involve a chance
of about 50% of estimating the completely correct tree structure and on average require less than one interchange between
neighboring populations to convert the estimated into the
true tree.

It would seem that in the case of fifteen populations an
average of four changes between the best estimated tree and
the true tree is not entirely satisfactory. Obviously, an

increase in the number of characters would improve the situation, but again we rely on future research for giving us an order of magnitude of the number of characters that can bring us nearer to a correct topology. It may seem strange that the method using the mean squared distances gives the best results in terms of time length, but is apparently not the best for selection of topology. We hope to be able to resolve this apparent paradox with additional data.

It is also worth noting that these trees provide a graphic representation of the information in a distance matrix, irrespective of any phylogenetic purport. The successive branchings of a tree represent qualitative hierarchical relationships, while the segment lengths reflect the quantitative aspects of those relationships. Numerical taxonomy often involves tree diagrams in this representational sense, and while we have not yet done so, we are aware that those methods could also be tested on our simulated trees.

SUMMARY

Methods of reconstructing phylogenetic trees have been compared by computer simulation. Earlier results on trees with four populations are briefly summarized. Results of new analyses in which evolution was simulated as a Brownian motion/Yule process for 6 and for 15 populations using in every case 20 independent characters are reported here. The methods being tested were used on the final positions of the points in the 20-dimensional character space and tested for their ability to reconstruct accurately the true evolutionary process which had been generated in the simulation procedure. A method of cluster analysis and the least squares method, both using the distances separating the populations, gave the most nearly correct tree with highest frequency, but a least squares solution using squared distances gave the best estimates of the true segment lengths. It was this last method which was expected to give the best results for estimating the evolutionary time elapsed since the split of the independently evolving populations. This emphasizes the importance of the choice of the appropriate measurement of genetic distance for results to be valid in terms of time of separation. In this paper no attempt has been made to discuss the importance of the other assumptions underlying the reconstruction of phylogenetic trees, of which perhaps the most important is the constancy of the rate of evolutionary change.

As a general conclusion, with 6 populations, 20 independent
characters do give a fairly good approximation to the true
tree when the assumptions of the theory are met. With 15
populations, understandably, 20 characters give rise to a
larger error. Further research is in progress to amplify
these results and cover other areas of the same general
problem.

LITERATURE CITED

CAVALLI-SFORZA, L. L. and A. W. F. EDWARDS. 1964. Analysis
of human evolution. *Genetics Today, Proceedings of the
XI International Congress of Genetics* 3:923-933.
CAVALLI-SFORZA, L. L. and A. W. F. EDWARDS. 1967. Phylo-
genetic analysis: Models and estimation procedures.
Am. J. Hum. Genet. 19:233-257, and *Evolution* 21:550-570.
COON, C. S. 1965. *The Living Races of Man,* Knopf, New York.
EDWARDS, A. W. F. 1969. Genetic Taxonomy. In *Computer
Applications in Genetics,* edited by N. E. MORTON, pp. 140-
142, University of Hawaii Press, Honolulu.
EDWARDS, A. W. F. 1970. Estimation of the branch points of
a branching diffusion process. *J. Roy. Stat. Soc. B.*
32:155-164.
EDWARDS, A. W. F. 1971. Mathematical approaches to the
study of human evolution. In *Mathematics in the Archae-
ological and Historical Sciences,* edited by F. R. HODSON,
D. G. KENDALL and P. TAUTU, pp. 347-355, Edinburgh University Press, Edinburgh.
EDWARDS, A. W. F. and L. L. CAVALLI-SFORZA. 1965. A method
for cluster analysis. *Biometrics* 21:362-375.
FITCH, W. M. and E. MARGOLIASH. 1967. Construction of phylo-
genetic trees. *Science* 155:279-284.
KIDD, K. K. 1973. Genetic approaches to human evolution. In
*Atti del Colloquio Internazionale sul Tema: L'Origine
dell'Uomo,* pp. 149-174, Accademia Nazionale dei Lincei,
Rome.
KIDD, K. K. and L. L. CAVALLI-SFORZA. 1971. Number of char-
acters examined and error in reconstruction of evolution-
ary trees. In *Mathematics in the Archaeological and
Historical Sciences,* edited by F. R. HODSON, D. G.
KENDALL and P. TAUTU, pp. 335-346, Edinburgh University
Press, Edinburgh.
KIDD, K. K. and L. A. SGARAMELLA-ZONTA. 1971. Phylogenetic
analysis: Concepts and methods. *Am. J. Hum. Genet.*
23:235-252.

KIDD, K. K. and L. A. SCARAMELLA-ZONTA. 1972. Relation-
     ships of domestic cattle breeds. In *Proc. XIIth
     International Conference on Animal Blood Groups and
     Biochemical Polymorphisms* (Budapest, 1970), pp. 241-
     244, Akademiai Kiado, Budapest.
KIDD, K. K. and F. PIRCHNER. 1971. Genetic relationships
     of Austrian cattle breeds. *Animal Blood Groups and
     Biochemical Genetics* 2:145-158.
MORTON, N. E. 1974. Bioassay of Kinship, this volume.
WARD, R. H. and J. V. NEEL. 1970. Gene frequencies and
     microdifferentiation among the Makiritare Indians.
     IV. A comparison of genetic network with ethno-
     history and migration matrices; a new index of genetic
     isolation. *Am. J. Hum. Genet.* 22:538-561.

!KUNG POPULATION STRUCTURE

Henry Harpending and Trefor Jenkins

*Department of Anthropology, Yale University,
New Haven, Connecticut 06520 and South African
Institute for Medical Research, Human Sero-Gen-
etics Research Unit, Johannesburg, South Africa*

Two currently popular approaches to the description and
analysis of local genetic variation in human populations may
be called the distance approach and the structure approach.

The genetic distance approach converts gene frequencies
into a set of "distances" among populations: increasing distances are assumed to indicate increasing evolutionary divergence. These distances are analyzed by the construction of
a cladogram which represents the history of the fissions a-
mong the populations which led to the observed distance matrix.
The cladogram may be constructed by one of several intuitive-
ly reasonable processes: maximum likelihood, least evolution,
or, most commonly in numerical taxonomy, a simple sequential
lumping process (this might be called the principle of minimum
computer time). Different algorithms may give quite different cladograms, but in general they are reasonable representations of the probable history and status of relations among
the populations.

For populations below the species level the tree model
is not an appropriate representation of population history.
Since genetic distance statistics can be written as functions
of population structure statistics and since there exist

This research was supported by the United States National
Institutes of Health (Grant MH 13611) and by the Clark Fund
of Harvard University.

models to predict population structure statistics from demographic history, the population structure approach seems to
be the more versatile and inclusive method of studying gene
frequency variation. Genetic distance studies seem now to be
limited to a more heuristic, rather than analytic, level of
description and comparison.

        Population structure may be defined, following MORTON,
as the effect of all parameters of non-random mating.   Information on population structure, then, may come from the
study of the demography of a population or from distributions of genes or gene frequencies over an area. In the former category are studies of parental and matrimonial distance,
social structure, pedigrees, isonymy, and migration matrices.
In the latter are phenotype bioassay (LI and HORVITZ 1953,
WORKMAN and NISWANDER 1968), mating-type bioassay (YASUDA
1968), phenotype-pair bioassay (MORTON et al. 1968, HARPENDING
1971), and what might be called WAHLUND bioassay (MORTON 1971).

        In this paper we report on a migration matrix approach
to the dynamics of internal gene-flow among !Kung hunter-
gatherers and on a WAHLUND bioassay of population structure
parameters from several marker loci. The statistics of population structure studies -- predicted from the demography
and estimated from the distribution of gene frequencies --
are coefficients of inbreeding and relationship. However,
there are various kinds of relationship coefficients whose
interrelationships are not always made explicit. We briefly
discuss these statistics and their interpretation before describing the population structure of the !Kung.

                              THE MODEL

        The conceptual model of the migration matrix approach
is of a large population divided into smaller units called
subpopulations. These subpopulations exchange members each
generation and then mate at random. The exchange among them
is described by a matrix $\underline{M}$ which has in its i,jth position
the portion of the genes of subpopulation j which come from
subpopulation i each generation. This matrix is assumed to
be constant from generation to generation, and its entries
are fixed proportions, not random variables. The migrants
are assumed to be a random sample of the inhabitants of their
subpopulation of origin.

This population undergoes genetic drift each generation by binomial sampling of the parental gametes. Fixation is prevented by linear systematic pressure which is assumed to be immigration from an effectively infinite outside population. The assumption that long-range migration, rather than selection, mutation, etc., is the agent of systematic pressure is necessary in order for all alleles to be described by the same model. Under selection, for example, the systematic pressure would be different for each allele.

We consider an autosomal locus with alleles A and a. In the infinite outside population the gene frequency of A is constant in time and it may be denoted by an unadorned p. The frequency of a is then q = (1-p). Each subpopulation receives a proportion s of its members each generation from this outside population, and these immigrants have a frequency of gene A which is p exactly, not a binomial sample from their population of origin.

These assumptions are a compromise between algebraic convenience and biological realism. This definition of systematic pressure is not readily interpretable in terms of ordinary demographic information, since even for an island receiving a known proportion of its members from a continental population the immigrants will be a random, rather than deterministic, sample, and a count of immigrants will not be a realistic estimate of s. Ordinarily, in field studies, systematic pressure is not readily ascertainable and, in applying the model, it is a nuisance parameter. Some empirical experience indicates that variation in s does not have a large effect on gene frequency variation within a population if the local inbreeding within the population is low. As the migration matrix approaches the identity matrix systematic pressure becomes important in predicting local variation. For example, for the !Kung we have calculated relationship coefficients using values of s of .01 and .10, and we find that they do not differ very much.

Given these assumptions one may calculate a symmetric matrix of coefficients of relationship among the subpopulations. Similar formulae have been given by IMAIZUMI et al. (1970), BODMER and CAVALLI-SFORZA (1968), and SMITH (1968). We would recommend that SMITH be consulted for an explanation of the model and that IMAIZUMI et al. be consulted for the correct algorithm. It is the relationship between the model presented by these authors and empirical variances and

covariances which we wish to discuss, as well as some minor
adaptations of our model to account for our field situations,
which may be of interest because it is typical of the situations studied by anthropologists.

THE INITIAL POPULATION

The model starts with K isolates all with gene frequency
p at a locus, i.e., the population is initially homogeneous.
SMITH (1968) interprets this to mean that local subpopulation
i of (census) size $w_i N$ is a binomial sample from a large population, so that its initial gene frequency before drift is a
random variable p_i with

$$E(p_i) = p$$

and

$$Var(p_i) = \frac{p(1-p)}{2w_i N} \qquad .$$

IMAIZUMI et al. (1970) take their homogeneity straight and take
an initial population with each subpopulation having gene frequency

$$p_i = p \quad (all \ i) \quad .$$

We take the initial K subpopulations as random samples
without replacement from an initial population of size N con-
taining 2Np $\underline{A}$ alleles randomly distributed. This initial
hypergeometric variation may be described by a K × K matrix
with diagonal elements

$$Var^{(0)}(p_i) = \frac{p(1-p)(1-w_i)}{2w_i N - 1}$$

and off-diagonal elements

$$Cov^{(0)}(p_i, p_j) \cong \frac{-p(1-p)}{2N}$$

where the superscript denotes generation. If

$$\phi_{i,j} = \frac{Cov(p_i, p_j)}{p(1-p)}$$

the initial covariance matrix may be written

$$\underline{V}^{(0)} = p(1-p)\Phi^{(0)}$$

where Φ is the relationship matrix.

RELATIONSHIP COEFFICIENTS

It is convenient that all variances and covariances in this model have $p(1-p)$ in the numerator, and that all derivations are independent of the initial gene frequency p. This means that, under drift and equivalent pressures, all loci should be subject to the same population structure and yield equivalent estimates of relationship coefficients. By relationship coefficient we mean the covariance (or variance) around an expectation p, divided by pq; that is,

$$\phi_{ij} = E\left[\frac{(p_i - p)(p_j - p)}{p(1-p)}\right]$$

where the subscripts refer to subpopulations i , j. Note that p, as used here, is not ordinarily ascertainable.

This definition is important, as will be evident further on, because there are various kinds of "inbreeding" and "relationship" coefficients and various kinds of variances and covariances which refer, respectively, to different base populations and different expectations of gene frequencies.

With M, the matrix of migration frequencies described above, with a diagonal matrix $\underline{U}^{(k)}$ which in its ith diagonal position has

$$\frac{1 - \phi_{ii}^{(k-1)}}{2N_i^e}$$

where N_i^e is the drift effective size of the ith subpopulation, and with a value for the systematic pressure, the series

$$\Phi^{(t)} = \sum_{k=1}^{t} (1-s)^{2k} \underline{M}^k U^{(k)} \underline{M}'^k \tag{0}$$

converges to a matrix Φ (IMAIZUMI et al. 1970).

SMITH (1968) gives an approximation to this formula, but the matrix corresponding to $\underline{U}$ has $1/2N_i^e$ on the diagonal instead of the more exact expression given by IMAIZUMI et al. (1970). The difference is not great, but with electronic computers there is no reason to use the approximation. The more exact form may be justified as follows. At reproduction each subpopulation's gene frequency in the new generation is a random variable with variance $p_i q_i / 2N_i^e$. The expected value of this variance is $pq(1 - \phi_{ii})/2N_i^e$, so the variance is decreased by a factor of

$$(1 - \phi_{ii}^{(k-1)})$$

at generation K; this correction is small (see KENDALL and STUART 1969, p. 127 [The results reported in this paper were calculated by the approximation and not by the exact method.]).

The matrix Φ or some statistic derived from it seems to be a natural measure of the amount of genetic drift to which a population has been subject. Two natural measures are the average relationship (or random kinship)

$$\sum_{i,k} w_i w_k \phi_{ik}$$

and the average inbreeding coefficient $\sum_i w_i \phi_{ii}$. We now discuss statistics derived from observed gene frequency variation and their relationship to these ϕ coefficients. We show that, in fact, the accuracy of this model is impossible to evaluate since sample statistics do not contain information about these parameters but only about some function of them.

REAL POPULATIONS

We write r_{ij} for the empirical sample coefficient of relationship between subpopulations i and j, that is:

$$r_{ij} = \frac{(p_i - \bar{p})(p_j - \bar{p})}{\bar{p}(1-\bar{p})} \qquad (\bar{p} = \sum_k w_k p_k) \qquad (1)$$

for any allele. For systems with multiple alleles the formulae given by MORTON (1971) are appropriate. In this section we assume that complete samples are available from every subpopulation and that gene frequencies are given by gene counting. That is, the matrix of coefficients $R = r_{ij}$ is regarded as known without error. The effects of uncertainty in gene frequency estimation, the bias induced by this uncertainty, and appropriate corrections are discussed in Appendix 2. Since the values r_{ij} are statistics it is natural to examine their expected values. First we define random kinship

$$\bar{\phi} = \sum_{ik} w_i w_k \phi_{ik} \quad ,$$

and random kinship of the ith subpopulation,

$$\bar{\phi}_i = \sum_k w_k \phi_{ik} \quad .$$

Of course,

$$\bar{\phi} = \sum_i w_i \bar{\phi}_i \qquad (2)$$

Then, we show in Appendix 1 that

$$E(r_{ij}) \cong \frac{\phi_{ij} + \bar{\phi} - \bar{\phi}_i - \bar{\phi}_j}{1-\bar{\phi}} \tag{3}$$

assuming that the hypergeometric or binomial sampling variance is included in ϕ. If the subpopulations are of equal size and arranged in a circle or some regular geometric figure so that

$$\bar{\phi}_i = \bar{\phi}_j = \bar{\phi} \quad \text{(all i,j)}$$

then (3) becomes

$$E(r_{ij}) = \frac{\phi_{ij} - \bar{\phi}}{1 - \bar{\phi}} \tag{4}$$

which is the form of WRIGHT's hierarchical population structure. Equation (4) is only true in general when statistics of subpopulation may be regarded as independent and identically distributed. (Equations (3) and (4) show that in real populations there is no simple relationship between genealogical inbreeding and non-randomness of mating or deviations from Hardy-Weinberg genotype proportions.) This may occur when all subpopulations are of identical size and do not exchange migrants, or when they exchange migrants in a circle or some other regular geometric arrangement. Equation (4) also holds for Wahlund F, $\sum_i w_i r_{ii}$, because of (2).

For the !Kung data, (4) is not a good approximation to (3). Further, random kinship and random kinship of subpopulations are not ascertainable from gene frequency data; this means that the model described here predicts what the r matrix should look like, but the reverse passage is not possible. (Given the definition of r_{ij} in (1), a little algebra readily shows that sample random kinship, $\sum_{i,k} w_i w_k r_{ik}$, is equal to zero, and that for any subpopulation i, $\bar{r}_i = \sum_k w_k r_{ik}$ is also zero.)

This is all relevant to some recent attempts to fit the model of MALECOT to several human populations (AZEVEDO et al. 1969). These authors have assumed that

$$\phi(d) = ae^{-bd}$$

and have estimated the regression parameters, a and b.
Apart from reservations about the algebraic validity of the
"phenotype pair bioassay" method (HARPENDING 1971), it is
clear that any solution to a likelihood system expressed in
terms of local gene frequencies measures what we call r and
not the values of φ predicted by MALECOT. (More exactly it
measures r plus non-random mating within subpopulations,
Wright's F_{IS}, which the Wahlund approach ignores, [BARRAI
1971]). Because estimates of φ(d) were negative at large
distances they fit an equation of the form of (4) using L,
the negative intercept of the fitted exponential curve, as,
in effect, an estimator of φ. Not only is this L not any
kind of estimator of φ, but (3) shows that scalar correction
for all distance classes is inappropriate. Populations on
the edge of an area will have lower random kinship with the
total sample than will central populations, so φ(d) at large
distances will be underestimated.

Our conclusion that there is no estimate of the matrix
Φ is not particularly discouraging, because this matrix is
not really what we desire in comparing gene frequency variation within various populations. The relationship coefficients measure total variance away from some unknowable equilibrium, not the local effects or subdivision or other aspects of population structure. A completely isolated, ran-
dom-mating island might have a high value of φ̄. But this
would not be of interest if we were interested in the population structuring within the island, and in comparing the internal structure on an island with that on another island.

This implies that we desire a science of comparative R
matrices rather than a science of comparative Φ matrices.
The natural summary statistic of an R matrix is "WAHLUND F"
which is $\sum w_i r_{ii}$ -- the gene frequency variance divided by
p̄q̄. This Wahlund F is related to average inbreeding by (4)
because of (2), that is, it differs by a scalar from the
total inbreeding measured by $\sum w_i \phi_{ii}$. But Wahlund coefficients from diverse populations will be heavily influenced
by at least two extraneous factors, the sample size, and the
manner in which subpopulations are chosen or defined. Because of this, we feel that there is still not a completely
satisfactory basis for comparing the population structure of
various populations of the world, although further analysis
of the effects of various partitionings of a population and

of changes in sample size might allow such a satisfactory
theory to be developed. (The equivalence between phenotype
bioassay and Wahlund bioassay is apparent with the more exact formula for Wahlund bioassay:

$$\frac{\sigma_p^2}{\bar{p}(1-\bar{p})} = F + \frac{1-F}{2N}$$

where the second term is mixed binomial sampling variance.
With subpopulations of size 1 this gives

$$\sigma_p^2 = \frac{1+F}{2} \quad .$$

Computing the variance directly as $\sigma_p^2 = \sum_i w_i p_i^2 - \bar{p}^2$ we have

$(p^2 + pqf) \times 1 + (2pq(1-f))(1/4) - \bar{p}^2 = \frac{1+F}{2}$.)

MIGRATION STUDY

The !Kung are hunter-gatherers living in the Northern
Kalahari desert in Botswana and Southwest Africa. They are
described by MARSHALL (1960), THOMAS (1959) and LEE (1965),
and they are the subject of several well known films by
JOHN MARSHALL. The !Kung included in this study are shown
in FIGURE 1. The numbered areas correspond to the subpopulations used in the construction of the matrix of estimated
migration frequencies. These areas are almost arbitrary,
since there is no perceptible clustering of social or breeding relations into isolates or semi-isolates. The migration
frequencies were calculated excluding data on movement within the last twenty years. Since then there has been movement of Bantu-speaking pastoralists into the area in Botswana
and many !Kung in Southwest Africa have settled at a station
set up by the South African Government. We feel that predictions from migration are good only to an order of magnitude, so we have not used the model to attempt to predict
the results of the disruptions of the last twenty years.
Instead, we constructed a migration matrix which we feel is
characteristic of the long-term !Kung patterning. Because
of the recent cultural disruptions and because we were unable to work in Southwest Africa, the subpopulations from

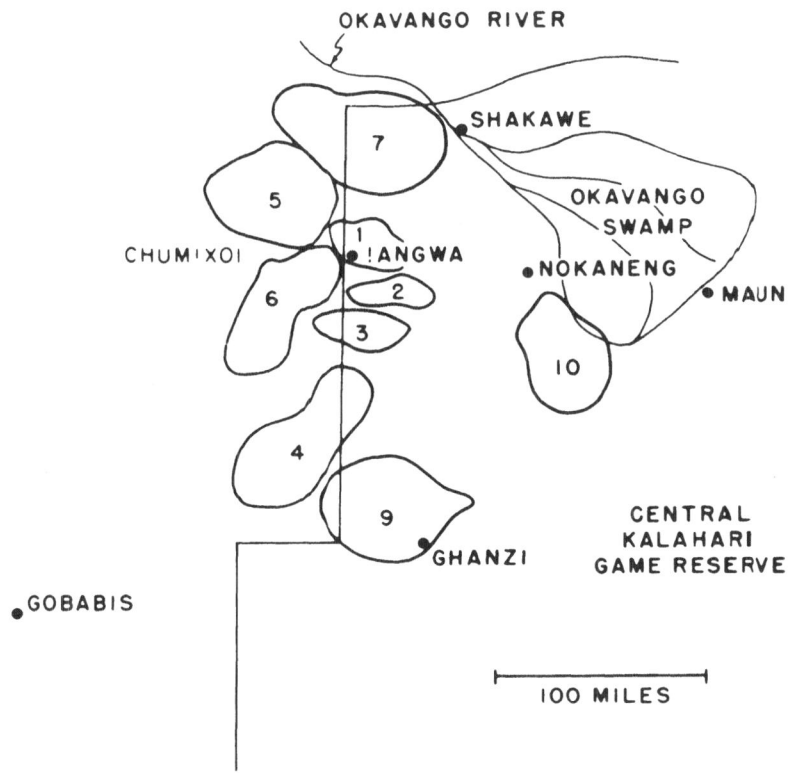

FIGURE 1.   Areas used in migration study.

which genetic samples were taken and those of the migration
matrix are not exactly the same.

     The counts of parent-offspring migratory events are
shown in TABLE I.   This table was the primary, but not the
only, source for the estimated migration matrix of TABLE II.
These counts refer only to birthplaces of adult fertile members of the population and their parents, so all these movements occurred well before the present Bantu and European
intrusions.   The matrix of counts was made symmetric by
guess in some cases, since for several areas wholly in
Southwest Africa, we have almost no information about
movement among them.

TABLE I

COUNTS OF PARENT-OFFSPRING MIGRATIONS

Area	1	2	3	4	5	6	7	9	10	Estimated Census Sizes
1	45	2	0	0	0	3	9	0	9	200
2	6	16	14	0	5	1	2	1	14	100
3	7	8	40	5	7	3	1	1	1	200
4	0	5	10	19	0	2	0	3	0	300
5	6	0	0	0	40	13	2	0	3	500
6	14	10	5	2	10	40	3	0	1	600
7	10	0	0	0	1	2	48	0	1	500
9	3	1	2	9	1	2	0	29	2	500
10	1	3	2	0	0	0	0	0	9	100

TABLE II

MIGRATION MATRIX: OLDER GENERATION
(Recent population movement effects removed)

	1	2	3	4	5	6	7	9	10
1	.556	.074	.041	0	.047	.125	.152	.009	.113
2	.050	.196	.149	.073	.046	.075	.030	.009	.182
3	.037	.204	.541	.195	.046	.063	.015	.017	.023
4	0	.056	.108	.463	0	.025	0	.076	0
5	.037	.056	.041	0	.615	.150	.031	.008	.023
6	.123	.111	.067	.049	.185	.500	.030	.017	.023
7	.123	.037	.013	0	.031	.025	.727	0	.023
9	.012	.018	.027	.220	.015	.025	0	.847	.845
10	.062	.148	.013	0	.015	.012	.015	.017	.568

TABLE III

PREDICTED RELATIONSHIP MATRIX $(x10^4)$
Systematic pressure = .01

309	275	271	281	296	317	356	330	336
275	296	294	298	297	313	335	337	353
271	294	318	315	299	315	333	346	329
281	298	135	350	314	331	350	406	343
296	297	299	314	345	346	369	369	350
317	313	315	331	346	365	387	387	368
356	335	333	350	369	387	471	414	402
330	337	346	406	369	387	414	545	406
336	353	329	343	350	368	402	406	408

TABLE IV

EXPECTED VALUES OF SAMPLE RELATIONSHIP STATISTICS $(x10^4)$
Systematic pressure = .01

42	8	0	−13	0	6	11	−32	10
8	30	24	5	2	3	−9	−25	28
0	24	44	18	0	1	−15	−20	−1
−13	5	18	30	−8	−6	−22	17	−10
0	2	0	−8	21	7	−4	−22	−4
6	3	1	−6	7	11	−2	−19	−2
11	−9	−15	−22	−4	−2	48	−26	−2
−32	−25	−20	17	−22	−19	−26	88	−15
10	28	−1	−10	−4	−2	−2	−15	95

Using M of Table II and one fourth of the census sizes given there as estimates of effective population size, we calculated the sum (0) for s = .01 until the result was stable to four significant figures. This matrix was then converted to estimates of R by equation (3). These two matrices are given in Tables III and IV, and r as a function of the distance between the subpopulations is shown in FIGURE 2.

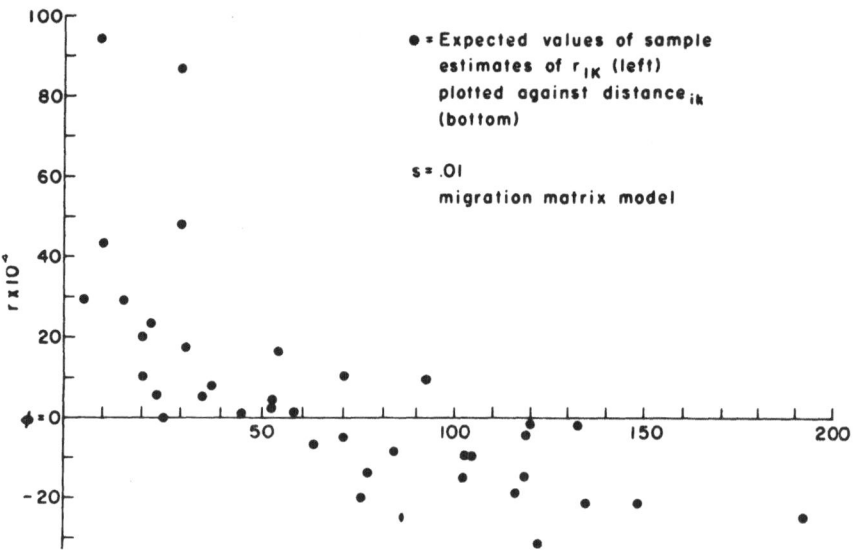

FIGURE 2.   Estimates of r as a function of distance.

GENE FREQUENCY STUDY

FIGURE 3 shows the areas studies. We have only completed tabulations for Rh, ABO, MNSs, Hp and Tf. The maximum like-lihood estimates of the local gene frequencies for each of the nine subpopulations are given in TABLE V together with the estimated sample and census sizes for each area. (That the approximate formula we used is unsatisfactory is demon-strated in TABLE III where some off-diagonal elements are greater than corresponding diagonal elements. Thus TABLE III gives ϕ_{11} = .0309 and ϕ_{19} = .0336, a result which makes little sense.) A matrix R was computed separately for each allele and these were simply averaged to form the overall

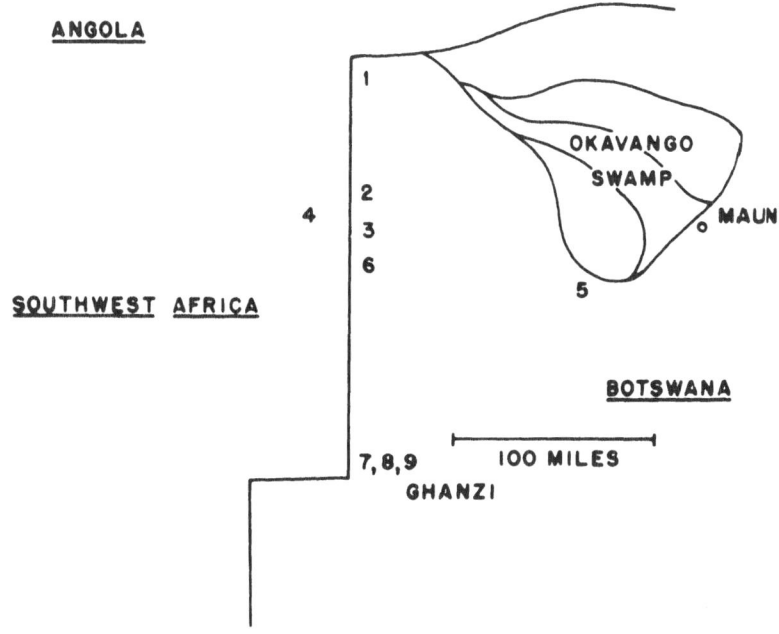

FIGURE 3.   Areas of the gene frequency study.

matrices given in TABLES VI and VII.   An averaging procedure
weighting each locus by degrees of freedom may be more appropriate, but we found very little difference between the two
procedures.

     These procedures were done on the whole sample and a
subsample of six populations, excluding the groups labelled
Mixed, Naron, and Cum!xoi.   The Naron are a Bushman group
living on the South of the !Kung and speaking a completely
unrelated language.   In Ghanzi, now a center of European-
owned cattle ranches, there is considerable mixture between
the two tribes and those villages which could not clearly be
given a tribal label were called Mixed.   Cum!xoi was excluded from the second tabulation because of the small sample
size.   Together with the large census size of this area, the
small sample size introduces large sampling error into the
estimates of $\bar{p}$ for every allele.   The six population subsample, then, represents "pure" !Kung.

TABLE V

GENE FREQUENCIES AND DEMOGRAPHIC PARAMETERS

		CDe	cDE	cDe	$cd^u e$	cde	A	B	O	MS
1.	North	160	000	744	000	096	279	000	721	150
2.	!Angwa	062	006	688	096	148	326	023	651	173
3.	/ai/ai	052	011	765	086	086	247	026	727	048
4.	cum!xoi*	020	000	839	141	000	265	000	735	091
5.	Sehitwa	113	006	726	155	000	259	041	700	115
6.	/du/da	034	000	966	000	000	210	009	781	110
7.	Kau Kau	025	022	805	092	056	184	034	782	134
8.	Mixed*	037	012	730	143	078	235	006	759	134
9.	Naron*	016	011	755	055	163	174	026	800	163

		NS	Ms	Ns	Hp1	Hp2	TfC	TfD	census[1] (N_i)	sample[2,3] (S_i)
1.	North	059	408	383	357	643	822	178	200	102
2.	!Angwa	072	376	379	341	659	852	148	400	311
3.	/ai/ai	027	499	426	322	678	807	193	150	139
4.	cum!xoi*	031	453	425	179	821	777	223	1000	050
5.	Sehitwa	044	415	426	347	653	895	105	300	164
6.	/du/da	055	293	542	317	683	784	216	150	117
7.	Kau Kau	080	335	451	288	712	912	088	1000	320
8.	Mixed*	039	496	331	393	607	930	070	500	166
9.	Naron*	039	480	317	393	607	915	085	2000	154

N_i=5700 S_i=1523

[1] Approximate

[2] Fluctuate for various systems--these sample sizes are for ABO

[3] Then, for each group: $W_i = N_i/\Sigma N_i$, $C_i = S_i/N_i$ (see text)

* Populations excluded from 6 population study

TABLE VI

ESTIMATED R MATRICES $(\times 10^3)$

Six populations unbiased

	1	2	3	4	5	6
1	016	010	006	002	004	-009
2		010	003	-001	-013	-005
3			006	001	004	-004
4				006	-008	-001
5					030	002
6						000

TABLE VII

ESTIMATED R MATRICES $(\times 10^3)$
Nine Populations Unbiased

	1	2	3	4*	5	6	7	8	9
1	024	015	009	002	014	012	-007	-004	-003
2		003	003	-001	006	-006	-004	000	001
3			-004	015	005	008	-004	-003	-004
4				017	006	025	003	-006	-015
5					007	-002	002	005	-008
6						031	007	-016	-011
7							-005	-002	-001
8								-007	006
9									-003

RESULTS

FIGURE 4 shows the distribution of the Wahlund F estimates
given by the various alleles for the nine population sample,
with and without the removal of estimated sampling bias by
equations (1,2) of Appendix 2. The biased values for the six
and nine population samples are, respectively, .0135 and .0197,
while the unbiased values are .0067 and .0028. The agreement
of the corrected values with the prediction of the migration
matrix (about .0040 at a systematic pressure value of .01)
is remarkable. Since the nine population sample merges
whole tribes and gives these large weight the difference
between the unbiased values of .0028 and .0067 probably reflects the non-inclusion of subdivision within these large
groups (see census sizes of groups 4, 8, and 9 in TABLE V)
and so is an artifact of sampling. In this situation, of
course, there is no correct sampling scheme since any subdivision of !Kung must be arbitrarily imposed by the inves-
tigator. On the other hand, the migration study referred to
subpopulations of the order of magnitude of those of the six
population sample so this is the pertinent comparison. The
Wahlund F value given by bioassay is larger than that predicted by the migration matrix, although the significance of
the deviation is impossible to evaluate. The value of the
systematic pressure used in the migration study, .01, is

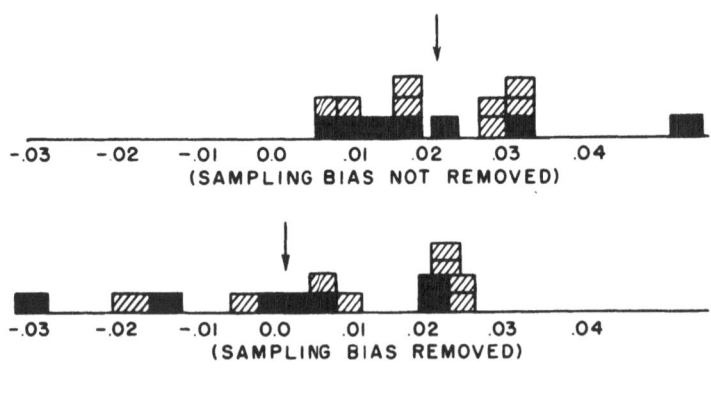

= Systems with dominant alleles: Rh, ABO

= Gene counting systems: MNSs, Tf, Hp

FIGURE 4. Nine populations – Wahlund F estimates.

completely arbitrary, but we note that the observed inci-
dence of Bantu admixture is probably lower than this figure
would indicate. The histograms show much more spread in the
Wahlund F values for the nine population study. The inclu-
sion of Cum!xoi with its large weight yet small sample size
must contribute much to this spread.

VARIATION OF F VALUES

If we accept the notion that the agent responsible for
maintaining the observed homogeneity of gene frequencies is
"long-range migration" (Bantu and Hottentot admixture), then
all alleles should provide estimates of the R matrix with
identical expectations. However, admixture now and certainly in the past has not been uniform among the subpopulations.
Populations on the periphery of !Kung land are more mixed
with their neighbors and there is much variety in the peoples
with whom the mixture occurs. They are primarily Hottentot-
speakers on the South and Southwest and Bantu-speakers of
many tribes on the North and East. This pattern of admixture leads to higher Wahlund F values than those predicted
by the uniform systematic pressure of the migration matrix
theory we have used, since the immigrants in different areas
come from parent populations with very different gene frequencies. For example, the Kau Kau intermarry frequently
with the Naron, and almost none of the other groups do.

The corrections for sampling bias given in Appendix 2
are minimum values; in the case of systems with dominance
the correction should probably be greater. FIGURE 4 shows
that gene counting systems seem to give more uniform F
estimates, while the extreme values are from systems with
dominance.

COMPARISON WITH OTHER PEOPLES

TABLE VIII shows the Wahlund F values of !Kung compared
with other areas of the world. The relevant comparison is
with biased !Kung estimates except for the Papago value
labelled unbiased. While the total population sizes and
the methods for choosing subdivisions in these various
studies are not comparable, the Bushman seem to be among
the least inbred of any of them. It is significant that

TABLE VIII

SOME WAHLUND F'S FOR SELECTED POPULATIONS

Population	F Estimate	Source
Parma Valley	.036	CAVALLI-SFORZA (1969)
New Guinea Tribes	.045	CAVALLI-SFORZA (1969)
Pygmies	.02	CAVALLI-SFORZA (1969)
Australian Tribes	.040	CAVALLI-SFORZA (1969)
South American Tribes	.082	CAVALLI-SFORZA (1969)
African Groups	.042	CAVALLI-SFORZA (1969)
Papago	.023	MORTON et al. (MS.)
!Kung Six Populations	.014	Present Study
!Kung Nine Populations	.020	Present Study
Greenland Eskimo	.005	WORKMAN (1970)
!Kung Six Populations (unbiased)	.007	Present Study
!Kung Nine Populations (unbiased)	.003	Present Study
Papago (unbiased)	.016	MORTON et al. (MS.)

the other populations with low F values, Pygmies and Greenland eskimos, are hunter-gatherers. There are good ecological reasons why hunter-gatherers should have this wide-rang-
ing outbred kind of population structure (HARPENDING and
YELLEN, in press). The advent of agriculture and settled
village life in human evolution probably brought with it a
major change in human population structure, a change from
a mobile and flexible social organization where any individual ranged over large areas in his lifetime to the fixed and
often more rigid and endogamous social organization imposed
by agriculture. This is reflected in the amount of local
genetic variability of these populations measured by the
Wahlund F values in TABLE VIII.

Elements of the estimated six population matrix were
lumped into four classes and plotted against geographic distance (in miles) in FIGURE 5. In general there is a decline
of r with increasing geographic distance. There is of course
insufficient information to judge whether it is linear, exponential, or of any defined form.

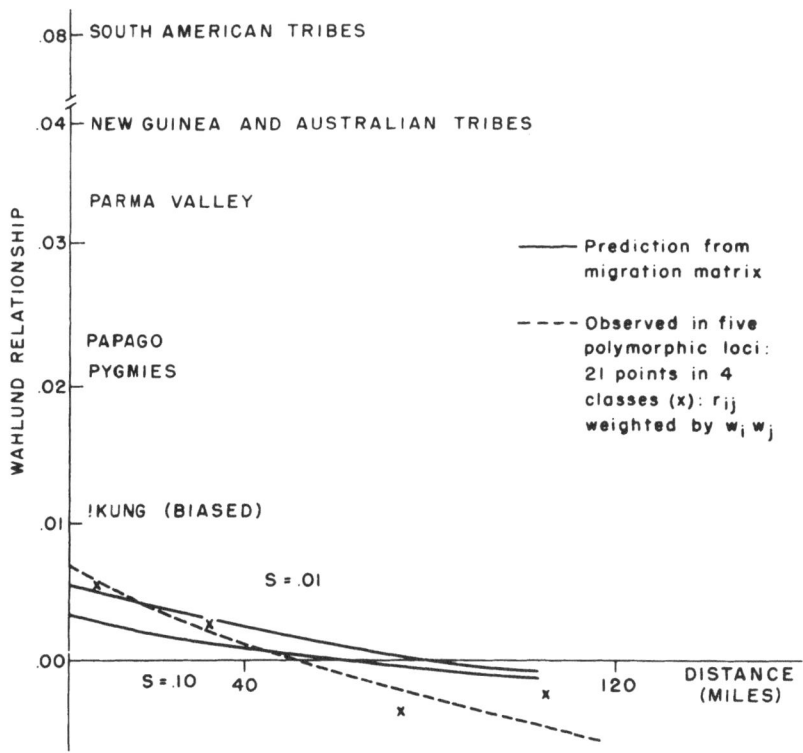

FIGURE 5. Estimates of r plotted against distance. Intercepts (Wahlund F) of other groups shown for comparison.

CONCLUSION

The patterning of local genetic variability among !Kung hunter-gatherers was studied by several methods. The observed frequency of gene flow among areas of !Kung habitation was used to predict the amount of variation which would accumulated under genetic drift. Gene frequency variation at five loci confirmed closely to prediction from the demographic model. A comparison of the estimated Wahlund inbreeding coefficient of the !Kung with those of other peoples shows the !Kung to be less subdivided and inbred than many agricultural peoples of the world and comparable to two other hunter-gatherer groups -- Pygmies and Eskimos.

Problems in the comparative study of subdivision and drift in human populations are discussed. The notion of local subpopulation is not well defined for the !Kung and for many other populations. Approaches which study individuals, such as phenotype bioassay and phenotype pair bioassay, should ultimately be more useful for comparative population structure studies.

Appendix 1 derives the expected value of the sample relationship statistic for a pair of populations if the relationship around the a priori expected gene frequency is given. Appendix 2 covers bias in relationship estimates from sampling error and the appropriate corrections.

LITERATURE CITED

AZEVEDO, E. et al. 1969. Distance and Kinship in Northeast Brazil. *Am. J. Hum. Genet.* 21:1.

BARRAI, I. 1971. Subdivision and Inbreeding. Letter to the Editor. *Am. J. Hum. Genet.* 23:95-96.

BODMER, W. F. and L. L. Cavalli-Sforza. 1968. A migration matrix model for the study of random genetic drift. *Genetics* 2:565-592.

CAVALLI-SFORZA, L. 1969. Genetics of Human Populations. *Proc. XII Int. Cong. Genetics.* Tokyo. pp. 405-417.

CAVALLI-SFORZA, L. and W. F. BODMER. 1971. *The Genetics of Human Populations.* W. F. Freeman, San Francisco.

FRIEDLAENDER, J. S. 1971. Isolation by distance in Bougainville. *Proc. Nat. Acad. Sci.* 68:704-707.

HARPENDING, H. C. 1971. Inference in Population Structure Studies. Letter to the Editor: in press. *Am. J. Hum. Genet.* (September).

IMAIZUMI, Y. et al. 1970. Isolation by distance in artificial populations. *Genetics* 66:569-582.

KENDALL, M. G. and A. STUART. 1969. *The Advanced Theory of Statistics.* Volume 1 (3rd edition). Hafner.

LEE, R. B. 1965. *Subsistence Ecology of the !Kung Bushmen.* Thesis, University of California, Berkeley.

LI, C. C. and D. G. HORVITZ. 1953. Some methods of estimating the inbreeding coefficient. *Am. J. Hum. Genet.* 5:107-117.

MARSHALL, L. 1960. !Kung Bushman bands. *Africa* 29:335.

MORTON, N. E. et al. 1968. Bioassay of population structure under isolation by distance. *Am. J. Hum. Genet.*

20:411-419.

MORTON, N. E. et al. 1971. Bioassay of Kinship. (This volume).

SMITH, C. A. B. 1969. Local fluctuations in gene frequencies. *Ann. Hum. Genetics* 32:251-260.

THOMAS, E. M. 1959. *The Harmless People.*

WORKMAN, P. L. and J. D. NISWANDER. 1970. Population studies on southwestern Indian Tribes. II. Local genetic differentiation in the Papago. *Am. J. Hum. Genet.* 22:24-49.

YASUDA, N. 1968a. An extension of Wahlund's principle to evaluate mating type frequency. *Am. J. Hum. Genet.* 20:1-23.

YASUDA, N. 1968b. Estimation of the inbreeding coefficient from phenotype frequencies by a method of maximum likelihood scoring. *Biometrics* 24:915-935.

APPENDIX 1

The Expected Value of Relationship Estimates

Assume that local gene frequencies at a locus are known exactly for an array of subpopulations. The gene frequency in subpopulation i is p_i, and the overall mean is $\bar{p} = \sum_k w_k p_k$. Further, let the relationship matrix be $\Phi = (\phi_{ij})$ so that:

$$E[(p_i - p)(p_j - p)] = p(1-p)\phi_{ij} \qquad (1)$$

where p is the "equilibrium" value of the gene frequency as determined by the systematic pressure.

Then, the estimator of the relationship between populations i and j is

$$r_{ij} = \frac{(p_i - \bar{p})(p_j - \bar{p})}{\bar{p}(1-\bar{p})} . \qquad (2)$$

Writing this as a product of the numerator and the reciprocal of the denominator, and assuming that they are uncorrelated:

$$E[p_i p_j] = p^2 + p(1-p)\phi_{ij}$$

$$E[p_i \bar{p}] = E[\sum_k w_k p_i p_k] = p^2 + p(1-p)[\sum_k w_k \phi_{ik}]$$

similarly,

$$E[p_j \bar{p}] = p^2 + p(1-p)[\sum_k w_k \phi_{jk}] .$$

For gene frequencies not too far from .5,

$$E\left[\frac{1}{\bar{p}(1-\bar{p})}\right] \cong \frac{1}{p(1-p)(1-\bar{\phi})}$$

where $\bar{\phi} = \sum_{i,k} w_i w_k \phi_{ik}$ so that var $(\bar{p}) = p(1-p)\bar{\phi}$.

Combining,

$$E(r_{ij}) \cong \frac{\phi_{ij} + \bar{\phi} - \bar{\phi}_i - \bar{\phi}_j}{1-\bar{\phi}}$$

where

$$\bar{\phi}_i = \sum_k w_k \phi_{ik}$$

$$\phi_j = \sum_k w_k \phi_{jk}$$

APPENDIX 2

Bias In Estimation of the R Matrix

In less perfect circumstances, sampling error introduces bias to the estimates of the r values which must be removed. To emphasize that we are speaking of error of estimation of local gene frequencies we use the symbol e^2 rather than σ^2 for the sampling variance of the quantity denoted by the subscript. We assume then that local subpopulation i has a gene frequency p_i, and that we are using an unbiased estimator $\hat{p}_i$ which has sampling variance e_i^2.

Since we are considering the distribution of local gene frequencies around $\bar{p}$, the sample mean, we may write:

$$E(\hat{p}_i) = E(p_i) \; ; \; E(\hat{\bar{p}}) = \bar{p} \qquad (1)$$

Then, letting:

$$E(p_i^2) = \bar{p}^2 + \bar{p}(1-\bar{p})r_{ii} \quad \text{(by definition of } r_{ii}),$$

$$\qquad (2)$$

we have:

$$E(\hat{p}_i^2) = \bar{p}^2 + \bar{p}(1-\bar{p})r_{ii} + e_i^2 \qquad . \qquad (3)$$

The estimator of r_{ij} is

$$\hat{r}_{ij} = \frac{(\hat{p}_i - \hat{\bar{p}})(\hat{p}_j - \hat{\bar{p}})}{\hat{\bar{p}}(1-\hat{\bar{p}})} \qquad . \qquad (4)$$

Expanding this by (1), (2), and (3) above:

$$E(\hat{r}_{ij}) = [\bar{p}^2 + \bar{p}(1-\bar{p})r_{ij} + e_{ij} - E[w_i\hat{p}_i^2] - E(\hat{p}_i \sum_{k \neq i} \hat{p}_k w_k)$$
$$- E[w_j\hat{p}_j^2] - E(\hat{p}_j \sum_{k \neq j} \hat{p}_k w_k) + \bar{p}^2 + e_-^2] \times E(1/\bar{\hat{p}}(1-\hat{\bar{p}}))$$

since the numerator and the denominator in (4) are independent. It is approximately true that

$$E(1/\hat{\bar{p}}(1-\hat{\bar{p}})) = 1/(E(\hat{\bar{p}}(1-\hat{\bar{p}})))$$

if gene frequencies are much larger than their standard errors. For the terms in the numerator:

$$E[w_i\hat{p}_i^2] = w_i\bar{p}^2 + w_i\bar{p}(1-\bar{p})r_{ii} + w_i e_i^2$$

$$E(\hat{p}_i \sum_{k \neq i} \hat{p}_k w_k) = \sum_{k \neq i} w_k [\bar{p}^2 + \bar{p}(1-\bar{p})r_{ik} + e_{jk}] \quad .$$

Since

$$\sum_k w_k r_{ik} = 0 \qquad \text{(all i)}$$

and

$$e_{ik} = \begin{cases} 0 & i \neq k \\ e_i^2 & i = k \end{cases} \quad .$$

This becomes

$$E(\hat{f}_{ij}) = \frac{\bar{p}(1-\bar{p})r_{ij} + -w_i e_i^2 - w_j e_j^2 + e^2}{\bar{p}(1-\bar{p}) - e_-^2} \quad i \neq j \tag{5a}$$

$$= \frac{\bar{p}(1-\bar{p})r_{ij} + +e_{ii}^2(1 - 2w_i) + e_-^2}{\bar{p}(1-\bar{p}) - e_-^2} \quad i = j \tag{5b}$$

where e_-^2 may be estimated as

$$e_-^2 = \sum_k w_k^2 e_k^2$$

In the results reported in the test we have ignored the

error terms in the denominators above and simply subtracted the terms in heavy brackets divided by

$$\hat{p}(1-\hat{p}) \, ,$$

from our raw estimates to obtain approximations to unbiased estimates. Estimates of

$$e^2_{ii}$$

were taken as the diagonal elements of the inverse of the information matrix for each subpopulation, and multiplied by $(1 - c_i)$ by analogy with hypergeometric variance.

Two simplifications of the above formulae are of interest. First, under binomial sampling from many large populations with a gene counting system

$$e^2_{ii} \sim \bar{p}\bar{q}/2N_i$$

$$e^2_{-} \sim 0$$

$$w_i \sim 0$$

and

$$E(\hat{r}_{ij}) \cong r_{ij} + 1/2N_i \qquad i = j$$

$$= r_{ij} \qquad\qquad i \neq j$$

If the populations are of equal size, and if we put

$$e^2_{-} = \frac{1}{k} e^2_i$$

$$w_i = \frac{1}{k}$$

then

$$E(\hat{r}_{ij}) \cong \frac{\bar{p}(1-\bar{p})r_{ij} + e^2_i(\frac{k-1}{k})}{\bar{p}(1-\bar{p})} \qquad i = j$$

$$\cong \frac{\bar{p}(1-\bar{p})r_{ij} - (\frac{1}{k} e_i^2)}{\bar{p}(1-\bar{p})} \qquad i \neq j$$

and under binomial sampling

$$E(\hat{r}_{ij}) \cong r_{ij} + \frac{k-1}{2N_i k} \qquad i = j$$

$$\cong r_{ij} - \frac{1}{2N_i k} \qquad i \neq j \quad .$$

A COMPARISON OF POPULATION DISTANCE AND POPULATION STRUCTURE TECHNIQUES

Jonathan S. Friedlaender

Department of Anthropology, Harvard University
Cambridge, Massachusetts

A number of papers in this symposium have focused upon the relative theoretical merits of the "population distance" and "population structure" approaches to local human variation. The blood polymorphic, anthropometric, and migrational information collected from 18 south-central Bougainville villages are, at this date, the only data set analyzed by both sorts of techniques (FRIEDLAENDER et al. 1971, FRIEDLAENDER 1971), and the different applications illustrate in a practical way the different aims, as well as the different merits and problems, of the two approaches. Here I would like to review the different sorts of conclusions the techniques have provided, and then present some new analyses from the population structure vantage point.

First, a few words about the sample are in order. Bougainville (FIG. 1), the northernmost of the large islands of the Solomons, has been inhabited for a considerable length of time, at least for the last 2000 years, and possibly for 4 or 6 times that long (JOHN TERRELL, personal communication). The archaeological picture which is beginning to emerge (and this only for the last 3 or 4 hundred years) has the island divided culturally into at least two distinctive areas. The southern section has close cultural ties with the nearby islands to the south, while the northern cultures are rather distinctive in such basics as their axe types, whose affinities outside the island are not clearly established. The current distribution of languages on the island reflects this north-south split. In the interior, a southern and a northern

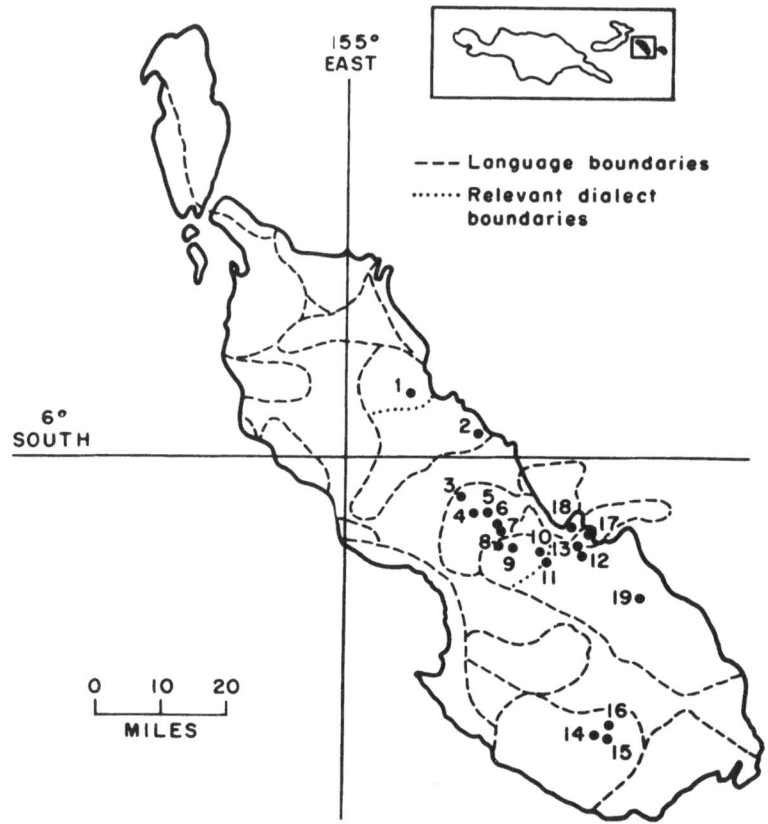

FIGURE 1.   Bougainville Island, Territory of New Guinea.
(The numbers refer to villages sampled.)

cluster of languages are quite distantly related to one another
(they share 5% of cognates in an abbreviated word list), but
their possible ties to other so-called Papuan (or non-Aus-
tronesian) languages outside Bougainville have not yet been
established (ALLEN and HURD). A third group has been
classified as a Melanesian language cluster, spoken primarily
by beach dwellers and sharing common ties with a number of
languages on nearby islands. It is not clear how long the
populations speaking these Melanesian languages have lived
on Bougainville, but there is little question that relatively
large scale movements have taken place along sections of the
coast as recently as 100 years ago. Traditionally the inhabitants of the island could nominally be described as tropical

gardeners tied to their land holdings, so that, relative to
hunter-gatherers such as the Bushmen, Pygmies, Eskimos, and
some Indians of the South American tropics, people in the
interior did not ordinarily migrate far from their places
of origin during their life-times. Although actual hamlets
and villages may be moved during a 10 or 20 year span, the
change in location is usually not one of more than a kilometer
or two. Also, as in other Melanesian groups, political ties
were traditionally weak beyond the hamlet or village level,
with no "tribal" level of organization, raiding between villages a common practice, and marriages ordinarily being con-
tracted between individuals living in close proximity to one
another (OLIVER 1955). Consequently, heterogeneity in gene
frequencies from one area to the next is extreme due to this
real subdividing of the population as opposed to the situation
which exists in ordinary shifting hunter-gatherer populations.

However, against this traditional pattern, Bougainvillians
have experienced a number of disruptive events in the last
50 years. First of all, in the early part of this century
when Germany and then Australia administered the island, hamlets in a given region were forced to merge into larger villages of approximately 100-200 people. Secondly, World War II
created grave hardships for the people and led to the temporary abandonment of many villages and garden plots, particularly in the south-western quarter of the island. Infant
mortality was extremely high (FRIEDLAENDER 1969). Many people
fled to the hills and then to the allied camp on the western
shore for food and shelter. However, even in northeast Siwai,
an area which was under direct assault, the great majority of
the surviving residents returned to their old lands and villages after the holocaust. Since the war, a general improvement in health conditions (most specificially the institution
of an effective malaria eradication program) and also the
breakdown in post-partem sex taboos, has led to a doubling of
the indigenous population. It is not clear that the proportion
of migrants from one village to the next has increased
(DONALD MITCHELL and EUGENE OGAN, personal communications),
but this would be expected.

With this description in mind, any application of the
population distance or structure approaches to the data must
be limited in its aims and sharply qualified. The current
array of villages in FIG. 1 hardly represents long-term sites
of populations which have remained undisturbed for even the
last 50 years, or the 100 years before that. Census sizes
have changed dramatically during the period we know anything

about. Health conditions have been sharply altered. And
since the time of this survey (1966-1967), many of the villages
in the sample have been even more seriously (and perhaps more
permanently) affected by the opening of a large strip mine
along the central mountain spine.

The blood polymorphism, anthropometric, and migration
data are therefore only a sampling of populations whose se-
parateness is vague and whose composition is constantly
changing. However, this is not to say, as some have claimed
for the more mobile hunter-gatherers, that village groupings
have no lasting importance or reference to time, space, or
population. Here people are more closely tied to their garden
plots, villages are conglomerates of old hamlets from the same
neighborhood, and transportation has been and is largely by
foot.

Using the population distance approach, we have constructed a number of different representations of the "distances" among populations (FRIEDLAENDER 1969 and FRIEDLAENDER
et al. 1971) of which two, utilizing the angular transform of
CAVALLI-SFORZA and EDWARDS on blood polymorphism gene frequencies, are presented here. The first "tree" (FIG. 2) is
derived from allele frequencies from seven blood polymorphisms
and the second (FIG. 3) is derived from an analysis of thirteen anthropometric measurements. Comparing the groupings
with the linguistic and geographic relations of the villages
given in FIG. 1, it is clear that even over this very small
area, 30 miles in extent, where so many disruptions have taken
place, the major divisions of the population in terms of language groupings and geographic separation are still reflected
in the biological variation over the area. While there are
minor variations in the local groupings of villages, the
north-south division around village 10 is clear in the blood
group and anthropometric trees, and the secondary linguistic
affiliations are also fairly obvious. While such general
conclusions as these are hard to contradict, it is a different
matter altogether to compare in a quantitative way the trees
or configurations derived from blood polymorphism distance
matrices, and the like. The trees, as gross simplifications
of the distance matrices, are quite far removed from the
actual data, and besides we know very little at this point
about the relevant distribution of tree lengths or how best
to judge levels of significance in such comparisons (see KIDD,
this symposium). In addition, the quantitative comparison of
the actual sets of distances is probably intractable, princi-

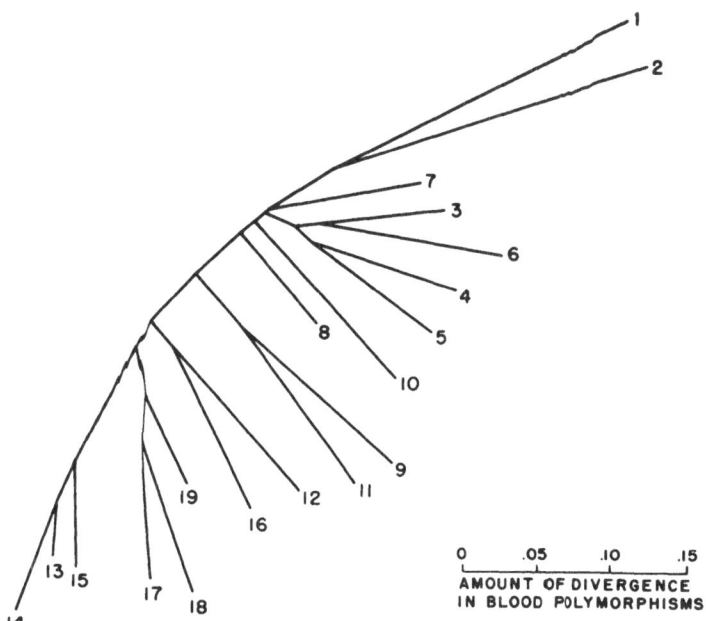

FIGURE 2.   Representation of distances among Bougainville
populations for seven blood group gene frequencies.

pally because the pairwise distances among all villages are
not independent and hence unsuited to most statistics which
measure relationship.   Nevertheless, these trees, with all
their obvious imperfections (or other representations of distance statistics), are the most useful results from the
Bougainville data analysis for students of the pre-history
of the area, or for those otherwise interested in similarities
of individual groups on the island.

In describing genetic variation within a population, many
biologists have become less interested in what they consider
the anecdotal results of population distance studies and have
turned their attention to the more generalizing approach of
so-called population structure analysis.   Here the concern is
with describing, and attempting to account for, non-random
mating within a population, either through an analysis of demographic variables or, more indirectly, through genotypic and
phenotypic ratios.

An appealing attempt to apply MALECOT'S theoretical model

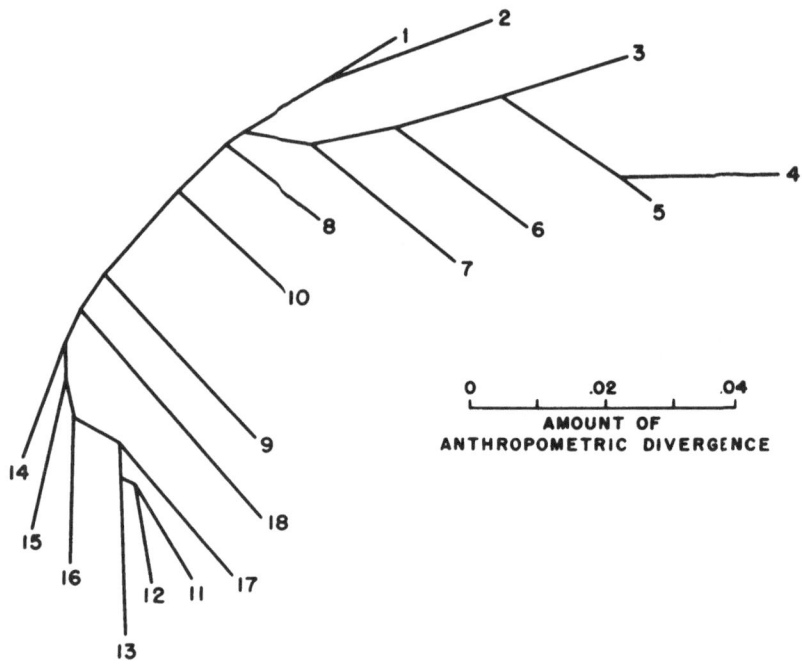

FIGURE 3.   Representation of distances among Bougainville
populations for thirteen anthropometric measurements.

of declining consanguinity or non-randomness over increasing
distance to human demographic and genetic data has been made
by N. E. MORTON and others (see MORTON, this symposium, and
especially MORTON, MIKI, and YEE 1968). The various techniques
MORTON'S group has developed over the last 10 years (embodied
in the computer programs ALLTYPE, DISTAN, NUMIX, BIOKIN, and
PHIT, described in MORTON 1970, and this symposium) can be
utilized to produce curves which attempt to describe the
average declining degree of non-randomness or similarity of
groups or individuals who are increasingly removed from one
another in space. Relationship curves of this sort, or their
parameters, should be comparable with respect to different

variables over the same population, and also with respect to
different populations in different continents. This compara-
bility of the statistics of population structure is an important advantage which is lacking in the population distance
approach, even though some distance and structure statistics
are functionally related. A previous attempt of mine at comparing the relationship curve derived from seven blood polymorphisms (FRIEDLAENDER 1971) with similar curves from previous studies (cf., IMAIZUMI and MORTON 1970) is illustrated
in FIG. 4. In this comparison, there seeems to be a clear
and satisfying dichotomy contrasting settled agriculturally
based village communities with more mobile and less fragmented
populations. However, such comparisons are not without their
problems. NEEL pointed out that the results for northeastern
Brazil and Japan in this graph do not seem reasonable, as
Japanese villages should have higher local variation gene frequencies than nordestino Brazilians. The fault undoubtedly
lies in the differences in the definition of the local breeding
unit, which was taken to be the prefecture in Japan, hence
undoubtedly underestimating local heterogeneity and the coefficient of kinship over the shortest distances. Valid comparisons, then, depend upon similarity in sampling techniques and
definitions. In all likelihood, bias in estimates may arise

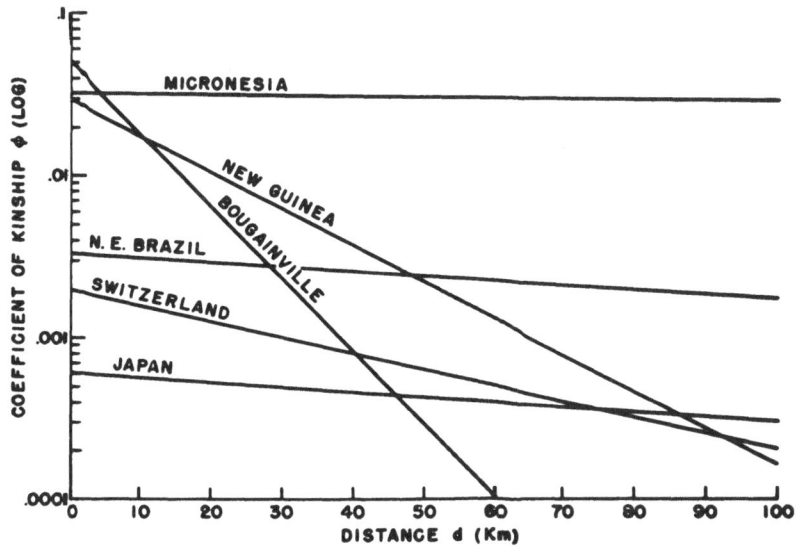

FIGURE 4. Relationship of kinship to distance.

from different sample sizes within the total population, differing arrangements of the subsamples in space, and lack of
subsample stability or identity either in the present generation or over time. HARPENDING (this symposium) has elabo-
rated on some of these difficulties, and has also pointed out
the weakness of the correction factor L. All in all, it is
clear that we are still not far advanced towards achieving the
sort of efficient comparative statistics we would like for
relationship curves. Nevertheless, in spite of his reservations, HARPENDING found good agreement between predicted relationship from his migration matrix and his own type of bioassay
of five blood polymorphisms in data collected from the !Kung.
He also concurs that settled, agriculturally based village
communities have extremely high local variation in gene frequencies, in his comparison higher than hunter-gatherers
(using Wahlund's F as the comparative statistic).

Here it seems appropriate to compare different measures
of population structure to the same population data and secon-
darily to see what sorts of differences arise using different
data from the same populations. For if we are to have any
confidence at all in our results, they must have some consistency within a population and in comparisons between
populations.

MIGRATION MATRICES

Because of the innumerable problems of accurate estimation
of the necessary input variables for a migration matrix (see
MORTON 1970 and HARPENDING, this symposium), I wanted to use
the simplest and most general approach I could devise. The
best solution seemed to be a hierarchical model. Two different
matrices were constructed, one dealing with short range migration (here defined as within language group migration) and
the second with medium range migration (here defined as among
language group migration). The medium range migration matrix,
or "among language" matrix, produced the following estimated
coefficients of kinship for pairs of language groups different
distances apart (following the method of MORTON et al., 1970).

Distance class	Mid-point	$\Phi(d)$
	km	
$d(0)$ = single language	10	0.02658
$d(1)$	15	0.01155
$d(2)$	28	0.00591
$d(3)$	38	0.00062
$d(4)$	49	0.00153
$d(5)$	69	0.00050

The short-range migration matrix, or within language group matrix, can be generalized over all villages in the sample in the following fashion. The matrix has 4 rows (for birthplace) and columns (for place of residence after marriage) where, for both rows and columns, the first element is the ith village, the second is the ith - 1 village, or adjacent village to the north, the third is the ith + 1 village, or adjacent village to the south, and the fourth element represents migration to or from other villages in the language group not included in the first three categories. The estimate of the effective population size was taken to be 0.2 of the 1963 census and the systematic pressure 0.07. The appropriate elements of the symmetric matrix of kinship coefficients can then be pooled to give average coefficients for the following comparisons:

Φ_0 = kinship coefficient of individual villages relative to their language group

Φ_1 = kinship coefficient for adjacent villages relative to their language groups

Φ_2 = kinship coefficient for pairs of non-adjacent villages relative to their language group.

The results, and the average distances for these comparisons, are as follows:

Distance Class	Assigned Distance (Km)	$\Phi(d)$
d(0)	2	0.02320
d(1)	5	0.00765
d(2)	8	0.00440

The two sets of kinship coefficients defined relative to different populations (village in language group and language
group in total sample) can be combined following familiar logic
to produce estimates of Φ for villages relative to the total
sample. For as the subdivision of the overall sample into
language groups contributes to the coefficient of kinship
among villages, the final vector of coefficients is defined
in the following manner:

Let Φ_L = average kinship coefficient of single language
groups relative to the total sample (here
$\Phi_L + .02658$)

Φ_T = short range coefficients corrected to reflect
language subdivision.

Then

$$\Phi_{T_0} = \Phi_0 + \Phi_L(1 - \Phi_0)$$

$$\Phi_{T_1} = \Phi_1 + \Phi_L(1 - \Phi_1)$$

$$\Phi_{T_2} = \Phi_2 + \Phi_L(1 - \Phi_2)$$

This produced the following table of combined estimates:

TABLE I

Combined Estimates Of Φ From Migration Matrices

Class	Mid-point	Φ(d)
	km	
d(0)	2	0.04916
d(1)	5	0.03403
d(2)	8	0.03086
d(3)	15	0.01155
d(4)	28	0.00591
d(5)	38	0.00062
d(6)	49	0.00153
d(7)	69	0.00050

The implication here is that language boundaries are quite important in restricting migration, and that, relatively speaking, they are as important if not more important, than local village groups in this respect. Whether or not this situation has existed longer than the past 30 to 50 years is doubtful.

BLOOD POLYMORPHISMS

With these predictors of relationship from migration data we compare different estimates derived from the seven blood polymorphisms, which have been previously analyzed by phenotype pair bioassay (FRIEDLAENDER 1971). In view of the controversy over the various estimation procedures proposed for the study of population structure, it is useful to compare results from different methods to gain some empirical notion of the range of variation of the estimates.

The three techniques used here are:

1) The phenotype pair bioassay previously utilized in FRIEDLAENDER (1971) and described in MORTON et al. (1968) where all possible pairs of the phenotypes of individuals in

the sample are generated and compared to expected values taken
from YASUDA'S mating type proportions. Phenotype pair bioassay
has been criticized on algebraic grounds (HARPENDING 1971)
and is currently out of fashion as an estimator of population
structure statistics. MORTON (1971) says estimates of Φ from
this method will equal $[F + 2y(d)]/3$ where $y(d)$ is the estimate
of the coefficient of kinship by the WAHLUND approach using
gene frequency variances.

2) MORTON'S BIOKIN essentially follows WAHLUND'S approach
and compares gene frequencies of subdivisions of the population with the population mean according to the following procedure: for 2 populations, a simplification of MORTON'S formula shows that;

$$\Phi_{ij} = \frac{1}{d.f.} \sum_k \frac{w_s \ (p_{ik} - \bar{p}_k) \ (p_{jk} - \bar{p}_k)}{\bar{p}_k} \tag{1}$$

where i = the ith population,

k = the kth allele,

d.f. = number of alleles minus number of systems,

and $w_s = \dfrac{N_i \ N_j}{N_i + N_j} \left[1 + v(s_h - 1) \right]$,

where N_i and N_j are the sample sizes and s_h is a measure of
the amount of information per individual furnished by the nth
system, and w is an "optimum weight estimated by BIOKIN"
(MORTON 1972) which in this study is taken to equal 1 for all
systems.
For the local group, or $d(0)$, a very close approximation is

$$\Phi_{ii} = \left[\frac{1}{d.f.} \sum_k \frac{w_s \ (p_{ik} - \bar{p}_k)^2}{\bar{p}_k} \right] \left[\frac{2N_i}{2N_i - 1} \right] - \frac{1}{2N_i - 1}. \tag{2}$$

For the local group average, this becomes

$$\bar{\Phi}_{ii} = \sum_i w_i \, \Phi_{ii} \, , \qquad \text{where } w_i = \frac{n_i}{N} \, . \tag{3}$$

3) "Unbiased Wahlund F" estimates have been introduced by HARPENDING (this symposium) to take account of bias in the above expression introduced by unequal sampling procedures, so that an unbiased estimate should be given approximately by

$$\Phi_{ij} = \frac{1}{\# \text{ alleles}} \sum_k \frac{(p_{ik} - \bar{p}_k) \, (p_{jk} - \bar{p}_k)}{\bar{p}_k \, (1 - \bar{p}_k)} \, , \text{ almost}$$

identical with equation (1) except for the weighting by alleles, and

$$\Phi_{ii} = \frac{1}{\# \text{ alleles}} \sum_k \left[\frac{(p_{ik} - \bar{p}_k)^2}{\bar{p}_k \, (1 - \bar{p}_k)} - \frac{1 - \dfrac{\text{sample}_i}{\text{census}_i}}{\text{sample}_i} \right] \tag{5}$$

and $\bar{\Phi}_{ii} = \sum_i w_i \Phi_{ii}$ as before. Aside from the differences in weighting, the results from (2) and (3) should be identical.

The comparative estimates for the Bougainville samples are presented in TABLE II. While in general the results from "phenotype pair bioassay" are lower than the gene frequency variance estimates, this is not always the case (see ABO) and there seems to be no consistency in the relationships. MORTON'S hypothetical 50% increase in estimation of local kinship from WAHLUND'S method does not materialize, as asserted by HARPENDING (FRIEDLAENDER 1971b). While an overall difference of .004 in estimation between "phenotype pair bioassay" and Wahlund F averages may seem insignificant, the major problem lies in the heterogeneity of estimates from the different polymorphisms. However, this heterogeneity does not blur the magnitude of the gross differences in kinship estimates of topical gardeners of the Pacific, hunter-gatherers, and societies with access to modern modes of communication.

In retrospect, these estimates are not widely divergent from the migrational parameters, where $\Phi_{ii} = .04916$, and in fact the unbiased estimate of Wahlund's $\bar{F}$ from blood polymorphisms are in excellent agreement.

TABLE II

COMPARISON OF ESTIMATES OF KINSHIP OR RELATIONSHIP FROM THREE
DIFFERENT TECHNIQUES OF BIOASSAY

System	Phenotype Pairs (DISTAN)	Gene Frequency Variances (MORTON'S BIOKIN)	Gene Frequency Variances with Sampling Correction (HARPENDING'S WAHLUND F)
ABO	.05998	.05450	.0510
Rh	.01592	.01261	.0088
Gm	.03114	.06406	.0743
IVN	.07252	.07534	.0777
Hp	.04778	.05530	.0554
PHs	.03349	.02976	.0383
Ss	.03836		.0416
MN	.02529		.0267
MNSs		.02593	
OVERALL	.04519	.04635	.0484

However, when the blood polymorphism data are subdivided
to reflect language boundaries as with the migrational data,
a different result is obtained. If language groups are taken
as the unit within which mating is at random, the estimates
here is Φ_L = .04008, or larger than the migration matrix data
would lead us to believe (Φ_L = .02658). Where villages are
taken as subunits relative to the language group, Φ_0 = .0232.
One possible interpretation, other than the likelihood that
the results are not strictly comparable, is that the current
migration matrix may underestimate the amount of isolation
which characterized the population structure of the island
(and which is still reflected in the blood polymorph heterogeneity). The proceeding discussion points up the difficulties
in estimation of local inbreeding or relationship relative to
the population of reference.

As one added observation, it is also plain from TABLE III

TABLE III

ESTIMATES OF THE AVERAGE KINSHIP COEFFICIENTS OF LOCAL VIL-
LAGES ($\bar{\Phi}_{ii}$), OF PAIRED VILLAGES ($\bar{\Phi}_{ij}$), AND OF THEIR OVERALL
AVERAGE ($\bar{\Phi}$), OR RANDOM KINSHIP

SYSTEM	$\bar{\Phi}_{ii}$	$\bar{\Phi}_{ij}$	$\bar{\Phi}$
Inv	.0753	−.00551	−.00023
Gm	.0641	−.00405	−.00023
Hp	.0553	−.00469	−.00025
ABO	.0545	−.00462	−.00023
PHs	.0297	−.00239	−.00043
MNSs	.0259	−.00215	−.00024
Rh	.0126	−.00116	−.00024

that little information is added by fitting curves to grouped
estimates of kinship coefficients for villages increasingly
removed from one another in space. The sum of all the elements
of the kinship matrix, $\bar{\Phi}$, must always approximate −1/(2N−1),
a sampling probability. Therefore, the higher the values of
local kinship, $\bar{\Phi}_{ii}$, the more negative will be the values of
the average kinship among villages, or $\bar{\Phi}_{ij}$. It is no suprise,
then, that in MORTON'S terminology as $\underline{a}$ increases, $\underline{L}$ and $\underline{b}$
become absolutely larger for a similar array of populations.
The points of interest are, first of all, a measure of local
inbreeding relative to some defined population and secondly,
if one is interested in the irregularities of the distribution,
the array of populations in a space determined by a principal
components analysis of the relationship or kinship matrix.

BIOASSAY OF TRAITS WITH COMPLEX MODES OF INHERITANCE

    If the problems of estimation in dealing with blood
polymorphisms are difficult, they are immensely compounded
when estimates of population structure statistics are calculated from traits with a complex mode of inheritance and
which are influenced by environmental variation. Yet it
seemed worth while to attempt this comparison as well.

    MORTON and GREENE (1971) have proposed one possible
treatment of traits of complex inheritance which could provide
comparable statistics of population structure. They use a
distance statistic which is a function of the coefficient of

kinship, which MORTON calls hybridity, θ.

If Φ_{ij} = probability that a gene in subpopulation i
is identical by descent with a gene in subpopulation j (an F_1 cross)

and Φ_{i+j} = probability that 2 genes taken at random
from a hybrid mix of i and j are identical
by descent (an F_2 cross)

then $\Phi_{i+j} = \dfrac{\Phi_{ii} = \Phi_{jj} + 2\Phi_{ij}}{4}$, as with the paradigm for

inbreeding in a family (MALECOT 1948). The hybridity coeffi-
cient θ compares Φ_{ij} and Φ_{i+j}, or the heterogeneity of an F_1
and F_2 cross between populations.

Since $\Phi_{ij} = \dfrac{H_o - H_{ij}}{H_o}$ and $\Phi_{i+j} = \dfrac{H_o - H_{i+j}}{H_o}$

we have

$$\theta = \frac{H_{ij} - H_{i+j}}{H_{i+j}}$$

and by substitution, $\dfrac{\Phi_{i+j} - \Phi_{ij}}{1 - \Phi_{i+j}} = \dfrac{\Phi_{ii} + \Phi_{jj} - 2\Phi_{ij}}{4 - 2\Phi_{ij} - \Phi_{ii} - \Phi_{jj}}$

which is zero when i = j and increases when i and j are more
distant. Therefore θ may be expressed as a function of kinship
and coefficients of current subpopulations (and their gene
frequencies). It should not depend upon the mean gene frequency of the array (as does ϕ) and hence MORTON'S statement
concerning its freedom from local gene fluctuations (MORTON,
this symposium). It is dependent, instead, on pairwise gene
fluctuations.

The values of θ vary proportionately to other measures
of distance, such as SANGHVI'S X^2 and KURCZYNSKI'S X_k, and the
like. For Bougainville, the average estimate of θ is .026
for the seven blood polymorphisms. It is this value which
serves as a comparative base for quantitative traits of complex inheritance.

In outline, MORTON and GREENE'S argument for quantitative traits with complex patterns of inheritance runs as follows. Under grossly simplified conditions (most especially where environmental effects are randomly distributed in the population),

$$\theta = \frac{\text{variance between } i \text{ and } j}{\text{total genetic variance}}$$

$$= \frac{D_{ij}^2/2}{2h^2T}$$

$$= \frac{D_{ij}^2}{8B+D_{ij}^2}$$

where $D_{ij}^2 = (x_i - x_j)^2 = 2$ x variance between i and j

h^2 is the heritability

T is the phenotypic variance in an F_2 cross between populations

B is the variance among sibships within populations

and in the same fashion,

$$h^2 = \frac{\text{genetic variance}}{\text{phenotypic variance}}$$

$$= \frac{8B + D^2}{4(W + B) + D^2}$$

where W is the variance within sibships.

Using these formulae, I have calculated estimates of θ and h^2 from different quantitative traits from the same individuals in Bougainville. Dermatoglyphics, particularly ridge counts, are known to have very high heritabilities (HOLT 1968), and the heritability estimates from this analysis of variance procedure are given in TABLE IV. They are arranged in decreasing order of their heritability estimates, with the four separate ridge counts all yielding considerably higher h^2 values, and, on the average, lower estimates of θ, although not as low as that estimated from blood polymorphs.

TABLE IV

ESTIMATES OF h^2 and θ from DERMATOGLYPHICS

Individual Ridge Counts	h^2	θ	Average θ
5th digit, right hand	.658	.026	
1st digit, left hand	.644	.041	.0385
1st digit, right hand	.616	.039	
5th digit, left hand	.559	.048	
Pattern types			
3rd digit, left hand	.466	.048	
1st digit, left hand	.464	.059	
2nd digit, right hand	.433	.051	
4th digit, left hand	.428	.048	
4th digit, right hand	.417	.043	.0476
1st digit, right hand	.416	.048	
5th digit, right hand	.414	.024	
2nd digit, left hand	.397	.050	
3rd digit, right hand	.391	.060	
5th digit, left hand	.241	.045	

HOWARD BAILIT has taken dental casts on approximately 1500 individuals from 14 of the same villages (excluding the Siwai and the smallest village in Nasioi) and has generously allowed me to analyze the dental measurements and observations from his study. The results are given in TABLE V, again arranged in order of decreasing heritability estimates. Again, there is a clear tendency for estimates of θ to increase with decreasing estimates of h^2, which is directly related to the changing ratio of B to D^2 for each parameter. The larger the ratio of B to D^2, the higher will be h^2 and the lower θ.

The estimation of θ and h^2 from anthropometric variables is even more unreliable because measurements were taken only on adult males, cutting down on the number of useful sibships (s = 404, n = 477). In any case, the results are presented

TABLE V

Dental Measurements -- Estimates of θ and h^2

Measurement	h^2	$\emptyset_s$	S
M^1 L-L	.805	.030	700
I^1 M-D	.804	.060	678
I_2 M-D	.744	.036	659
P^1 M-D	.721	.059	654
I^2 M-D	.701	.070	663
M_1 M-D	.700	.040	700
I^2 L-L	.699	.047	663
P^2 L-L	.691	.052	637
M_1 L-L	.683	.030	700
M^1 M-D	.665	.047	700
I^1 L-L	.642	.038	678
I_1 L-L	.633	.069	623
C^1 L-L	.627	.067	635
C_1 M-D	.626	.115	626
M^2 L-L	.597	.097	606
M_2 M-D	.560	.082	606
M^2 L-L	.536	.051	592
P_1 L-L	.531	.115	643
P_1 M-D	.530	.083	643
P^1 M-D	.522	.108	654
I_1 M-D	.518	.087	623
C^1 M-D	.506	.031	635
P^2 L-L	.506	.150	631
M^2 M-D	.484	.084	592
P^2 M-D	.448	.177	637
C_1 L-L	.369	.129	626
I_2 L-L	.359	.154	659
P_2 M-D	.240	.133	631

M-D = mesial-distal length
L-L = labio-lingual length

in Table VI.

TABLE VI

Anthropometric Estimates of θ and h^2

Measurement	h^2	θ
Nose Breadth	1.061	.069
Sitting Height	1.035	.053
Weight	1.024	.043
Stature	.959	.082
Nose Height	.879	.677
Chest Breadth	.801	.190
Arm Length	.735	.080
Head Breadth	.724	.312
Mim front br.	.714	.063
Bizygomatic br.	.665	.107
Head Length	.646	.257
Total Face Height	.637	.169
Bigonial br.	.585	.068

$$n = 477, \quad s = 404$$

These various attempts at approximating statistics which are presumably more efficiently estimated from blood polymorphisms are not satisfying in the end. They are much too heterogeneous to be useful or at all trustworthy. The heritability estimates for those traits with sufficient data are at least in the right ballpark, and those with the highest heritability are the traits which approach the θ value of the blood polymorphisms.

In conclusion, it seems that we have reasonable ways of describing blood polymorphism gene frequency heterogeneity within a population which, for this set of data, all provide consistent estimates. The average value is not inconsistent with migration estimates. However, attempts to derive statistics of population structure from traits of complex inheritance have so far been unsatisfactory.

LITERATURE CITED

ALLEN, J. and C. HURD. (N.D.) Languages of the Bougainville District. Summer Institute of Linguistics, Ukarumpa, New Guinea.

FRIEDLAENDER, J. S. 1969. Biological divergences over population boundaries in south-central Bougainville. Ph.D. thesis. Harvard University, Cambridge, Massachusetts.

FRIEDLAENDER, J. S. 1971. The population structure of south-central Bougainville. *Am. J. Phys. Anth.* 35:13-25.

FRIEDLAENDER, J. S. 1971b. Isolation by distance in Bougainville. *Proc. Nat. Acad. Sci.* 68:704-707.

FRIEDLAENDER, J. S., L. A. SGARAMELLA-ZONTA, K. K. KIDD, L. Y. C. LAI, P. CLARK and R. J. WALSH. 1971. Biological divergences in south-central Bougainville. *Am. J. Hum. Genet.* 23:253-270.

HARPENDING, H. 1971. Inference in Population Structure studies. Letter to the Editor. *Am. J. Hum. Genet.* 23:536-538.

HOLT, S. B. 1968. *The Genetics of Dermal Ridges.* Charles Thomas, Springfield, Illinois.

IMAIZUMI, Y. and N. E. MORTON. 1970. Isolation by distance in artificial populations. *Genetics* 66:569-582.

MALECOT, G. 1948. Les mathématiques de l'hérédité. Masson, Paris.

MORTON, N. E. 1970. Population structure. In: *Computer Applications in Genetics.* Edited by N. E. Morton, University of Hawaii Press, Honolulu, pp. 61-68.

MORTON, N. E. 1971. Inference in population structure studies. Letter to the Editor. *Am. J. Hum. Genet.* 23:538-539.

MORTON, N. E. and D. GREENE. 1971. Pingelap and Mokil Atolls: Anthropometrics. MS.

MORTON, N. E., C. MIKI and S. YEE. 1968. Bioassay of population structure under isolation by distance. *Am. J. Hum. Genet.* 20:411-419.

OLIVER, D. L. 1955. *Solomon Islands Society.* Harvard University Press, Cambridge, Massachusetts.

INDEX